PEDIATRIC FIRST AID, CPR, AND AED

Second Edition

National Safety Council

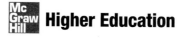 **Higher Education**

Boston   Burr Ridge, IL   Dubuque, IA   New York   San Francisco   St. Louis
Bangkok   Bogotá   Caracas   Kuala Lumpur   Lisbon   London   Madrid   Mexico City
Milan   Montreal   New Delhi   Santiago   Seoul   Singapore   Sydney   Taipei   Toronto

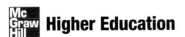

Higher Education

PEDIATRIC FIRST AID, CPR, AND AED, SECOND EDITION

Published by McGraw-Hill, a business unit of The McGraw-Hill Companies, Inc., 1221 Avenue of the Americas, New York, NY 10020. Copyright © 2008 from National Safety Council. All rights reserved. No part of this publication may be reproduced or distributed in any form or by any means, or stored in a database or retrieval system, without the prior written consent of the National Safety Council, including, but not limited to, in any network or other electronic storage or transmission, or broadcast for distance learning.

Some ancillaries, including electronic and print components, may not be available to customers outside the United States.

This book is printed on acid-free paper.

4 5 6 7 8 9 0 QPV/QPV 0 9

ISBN 978–0–07–319449–3
MHID 0–07–319449–2

Publisher, Career Education: *David T. Culverwell*
Senior Sponsoring Editor: *Claire Merrick*
Director of Development: *Kristine Tibbetts*
Editorial Coordinator: *Michelle L. Zeal*
Outside Managing Editor: *Kelly Trakalo*
Senior Marketing Manager: *Lisa Nicks*
Senior Project Manager: *Sheila M. Frank*
Senior Production Supervisor: *Laura Fuller*
Lead Media Project Manager: *Audrey A. Reiter*
Senior Media Producer: *Renee Russian*
Senior Coordinator of Freelance Design: *Michelle D. Whitaker*
Cover/Interior Designer: *Studio Montage*
Lead Photo Research Coordinator: *Carrie K. Burger*
Photo Research: *Pam Carley/Sound Reach*
Supplement Producer: *Tracy L. Konrardy*
Compositor: *Electronic Publishing Services Inc., NYC*
Typeface: *11.5/13 Minion*
Printer: *Quebercor World Versailles Inc.*

ISSN: 1932-5630

Photo Credits: Page 32, Page 34 top: Courtesy Bradley R. Davis; Page 34 middle: © Dr. P. Marazzi/Photo Researchers, Inc.; Page 34 bottom: © Custom Medical Stock Photo; Page 35, Page 50 top, Page 50 bottom: © Dr. P. Marazzi/Photo Researchers, Inc.; Page 51 top: Courtesy Bradley R. Davis; Page 51 bottom: © Dr. P. Marazzi/Photo Researchers, Inc.; Page 53, Page 63: © Mediscan; Page 84 top: www.poison-ivy.org; Page 84 middle: Courtesy Mario D. Vaden, Certified Arborist, www.mdvaden.com; Page 84 bottom: © Gilbert S. Grant/Photo Researchers, Inc.; Page 86 top: Centers for Disease Control and Prevention; Page 86 bottom: © Robert Noonan/Photo Researchers, Inc.; Page 87 top left: © Brad Mogen/Visuals Unlimited; Page 87 bottom: Photo by Scott Bauer, Agricultural Research Service, USDA; Page 88: © Caliendo/Custom Medical Stock Photo; Page 89: © DV13/Getty Royalty Free; Page 90 left: © Mediscan; Page 90 right: © SIU/Visuals Unlimited; Page 108 bottom left: CDC/J. D. Millar; Page 108 bottom right: © Dr. P. Marazzi/Photo Researchers, Inc.; Page 113: © Mediscan; Page 114: © St. Bartholomew's Hospital/Photo Researchers, Inc.; Page 116 bottom left, Page 116 bottom right: Centers for Disease Control; Page 117 bottom left: CDC/Dr. Lucille K. Georg; Page 117 bottom right: © Mediscan; Page 118 bottom left: © Dr. P. Marazzi/Photo Researchers, Inc.; Page 118 bottom right: © St. Bartholomew's Hospital/Photo Researchers, Inc.
All other photographs © National Safety Council/Rick Brady, photographer.

NATIONAL SAFETY COUNCIL MISSION STATEMENT
The mission of the National Safety Council is to educate and influence people to prevent accidental injury and death.

DISCLAIMER
Although the information and recommendations contained in this publication have been compiled from sources believed to be reliable, the National Safety Council makes no guarantee as to, and assumes no responsibility for, the correctness, sufficiency, or completeness of such information or recommendations. Other or additional safety measures may be required under particular circumstances.

www.mhhe.com

About the National Safety Council

Founded in 1913, the National Safety Council is a nonprofit membership organization devoted to protecting life and promoting health. Its mission "is to educate and influence people to prevent accidental injury and death."

The National Safety Council has been the leader in protecting life and promoting health in the workplace for over 90 years. With a vision of "Making Our World a Safer Place," the Council has helped make great improvements in workplace safety, and expanded its focus to include safety on the roads, and in the home and community. Working through its 48,000 members, and in partnership with public agencies, private groups, and other associations, the Council serves as an impartial information gathering and distribution organization; it disseminates safety, health, and environmental materials from its Itasca, Illinois, headquarters through a network of regional offices, chapters, and training centers.

In 1990 we established First Aid and CPR courses to promote effective emergency response. Since then, we have grown to meet the changing needs of emergency responders at all levels of expertise. Upon successful completion of this course, you join more than 10 million National Safety Council trained responders protecting life and promoting health.

Acknowledgments

The National Safety Council wishes to thank the following Chapters and individuals for their assistance in developing this program:

For providing technical advice and assistance with photography: Chesapeake Region Safety Council.

For providing technical advice and assistance with videotaping: the Arizona Chapter, National Safety Council, John Stubbs and C. J. Anderson.

For providing technical writing services: Tom Lochhaas, Editorial Services, Newburyport, MA.

Many National Safety Council staff and affiliates have contributed to the production of this book and we would like to acknowledge the following people for their assistance:

For reviewing and providing oversight of the content: Paul Satterlee, MD, National Safety Council Medical Director and Emergency Physician, North Memorial Medical Center, Minneapolis.

For providing vision and support: Donna M. Siegfried, Executive Director, Emergency Care.

For providing oversight of content and interfacing with McGraw-Hill staff on all areas of production: Barbara Caracci, Director of Emergency Care Programs and Training.

For providing marketing support: Donna Fredenhagen, Product Manager.

For providing day-to-day assistance: Kathy Safranek, Project Administrator.

Publisher's Acknowledgments

Steve Forshier, M.Ed., R.T. (R)
Pima Medical Institute
Mesa, AZ

Elizabeth Hennisse
Florida Metropolitan University
Orlando, FL

Beth Inbau, BS, NREMT
National Safety Council, South Louisiana Chapter
Kenner, LA

Brian Summers
Health Promotions
University of Texas at El Paso
El Paso, TX

Judith Tanner
Sacramento City College
Sacramento, CA

Emily E. Williamson
Family and Consumer Sciences Dept.
University of Louisiana at Monroe
Monroe, LA

Table of Contents

Introduction

Why Learn Injury Prevention and First Aid?

Injuries are the number one health problem for children in the United States. Injuries to infants and children vary from simple cuts and bruises to life-threatening emergencies. According to the National SAFE KIDS Campaign, following are the most common injuries leading to death in children at different ages:

Infants (0–1 years)

- Choking
- Motor vehicle occupant injury
- Drowning
- Fires and burns

Children (1–4 years)

- Drowning
- Motor vehicle occupant injury
- Pedestrian injuries
- Fires and burns
- Choking

Children (5–14 years)

- Motor vehicle occupant injury
- Pedestrian injuries
- Drowning
- Fires and burns
- Bicycle injuries

Each year more than six million children under age 14 are treated in emergency rooms for unintentional injuries. Tragically, about 5,000 children die every year from their injuries. Tens of thousands more have permanent disabilities resulting from their injuries.

COMMON CHILDHOOD INJURIES

- Falls
- Struck by/against
- Overexertion
- Bite/sting
- Cut/pierce
- Poisoning
- Motor vehicle occupant
- Bicycle injury
- Airway obstruction from foreign object
- Fire/burn

(Adapted from National Safety Council, *Injury Facts®, 2005–2006 edition*)

PREVENTING INJURIES IN CHILDHOOD

It has been estimated that 90% of all injuries to infants and children could have been prevented. Obviously, prevention is a better solution than simply being prepared to give first aid once an injury has occurred. For guidelines you can follow to prevent injuries and ensure that your childcare center, home, school, and other settings are safe for infants and children, see Chapters 14, 15, and 16 and visit www.nsc.org.

WHAT IS FIRST AID?

First aid is the immediate help given by an adult, usually a caretaker, to a child who is injured or experiences sudden illness, until appropriate medical help arrives or the child is seen by a healthcare provider. First aid often is not the only treatment the child needs, but it helps the child for the usually short time until advanced care begins.

Most first aid is fairly simple and does not require extensive training or equipment. With the first aid training in this course and a basic first aid kit, you can perform first aid.

Goals of First Aid

- Keep the child alive.
- Prevent the child's condition from getting worse.
- Help promote the child's recovery from the injury or illness.
- Ensure that the child receives medical care.
- Keep the child calm and distracted while providing care.

THE EMERGENCY MEDICAL SERVICES SYSTEM

People who are trained in first aid are the first step in the Emergency Medical Services (EMS) system. As a first aider you are *only* the first step, so part of your responsibility is to make sure the EMS system responds to help a child with a serious injury or sudden illness by calling 9-1-1 (or your local or company emergency number). You will learn more about calling EMS in Chapter 1. In most communities in the United States, help will arrive within minutes. The first aid you give helps the child until then.

BE PREPARED

- ***Know what to do.*** This first aid course will teach you what to do.
- ***Stay ready.*** A first aid situation can occur to a child at any time and in any place. Think of yourself as a first aider who is always ready to step in and help. You should always feel confident that you can help an injured or ill child.
- ***Have a personal first aid kit, and know where kits are kept in your childcare center, home, or other setting.*** Be sure first aid kits are well stocked with the right supplies. Keep emergency phone numbers, such as EMS, the Poison Control Center, and other emergency agencies, in a handy place.
- ***Know whether your community uses 9-1-1 or a different emergency telephone number.*** Note that this manual says "Call 9-1-1" throughout. If your community does not use the 9-1-1 system, call your local emergency number instead.

PREVENTING EMERGENCIES

Remember that many injuries can be prevented, and always take the appropriate steps to ensure that places where children are present are safe for them. Learn to be watchful for any hazards in the environment—do not wait for a problem to arise before acting to eliminate hazards and risks to children.

DISASTER PREPAREDNESS

Whether you are a parent or childcare provider, you should also be prepared in case of natural disaster and other incidents. In some states, such preparedness is required for childcare providers.

Childcare providers must be prepared for catastrophic emergencies such as earthquake, flood, and fire. Be prepared to evacuate areas, and know how to respond if basic services such as water, gas, electricity, or telephones are disrupted.

Childcare providers should have an action plan for these types of emergencies. This plan can be prepared with the assistance of local EMS, fire, and/or law enforcement authorities.

The Federal Emergency Management Agency (FEMA) provides these basic guidelines if a disaster occurs:

- Use flashlights, not matches, candles, or other open flames. Do not turn on electrical switches if you suspect damage.
- Sniff for gas leaks. If you suspect a leak, turn off the main gas valve, open windows, and evacuate.
- Turn off any other damaged utilities.
- Clean up any flammable liquids immediately.
- Have a plan that details your evacuation process and routes.
- Maintain a disaster kit that includes a supply of water, infant- or child-appropriate food, first aid kit, clothing, bedding, tools, emergency supplies, and special items such as individual medications. Keep the items that you would most likely need during an evacuation in an easy-to-carry container such as a backpack.

- Store water in plastic containers. Generally, children will need more than 2 quarts of drinking water per day.
- Store at least a 3-day supply of non-perishable food such as high-energy bars, or ready-to-eat canned meats, fruits, and vegetables.

If you are employed in a childcare center, you should know other guidelines required at your center.

YOUR FIRST AID KIT

A well-stocked first aid kit should be present in your home, vehicle, and childcare center. Take one with you on activities such as camping and boating. A cell phone is also helpful in most emergencies.

Ensure that the first aid kit is in a locked container kept where children cannot access it. In a childcare center, all adults should know where the kit is kept. The contents of the kit should be checked regularly, and all items should be replaced as used. Medicines taken by individual children should not be kept in the first aid kit but locked safely in another location.

Make sure your first aid kit includes the items shown in **Figure I-1**. Note that you may not

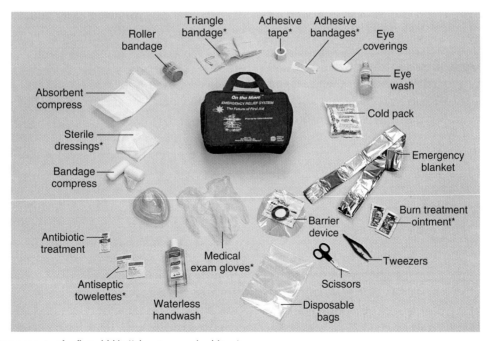

Figure I-1 Components of a first aid kit (*denotes required item).

necessarily use all items in a kit just because they are there. For example, first aiders other than a child's parents or authorized childcare provider generally do not give medications such as prescription or over-the-counter pain medication (such as acetaminophen).

In addition to these first aid kit items, other items may be required. In California, for example, first aid kits in childcare centers must include a flashlight with extra batteries, a pen, and paper. They may not include burn ointment.

LEGAL ISSUES

Can You Be Sued for Giving First Aid?

Generally you do not need to be concerned about being sued for giving first aid. If you give first aid as you are trained to in this course, and do your best, there is little chance of being found legally liable. To protect yourself, always follow these guidelines:

1. Act *only* as you are trained to act.
2. Have permission to give first aid.
3. Do not move an injured child unnecessarily.
4. Call for professional help.
5. Keep giving care until help arrives.

Must You Give First Aid?

In general, in most states you have no legal obligation to give first aid as a citizen or a bystander at the scene of an emergency. As the specific obligations may vary, ask your instructor about the law in your area. If you do begin giving first aid, however, it is important to note that you are obligated to continue giving care if you can and to remain with the victim.

In certain situations, however, you may have a legal obligation to give first aid. If you work as a childcare provider and giving first aid is part of your job, you have a legal responsibility to act appropriately. This is called a **duty to act.** If you are employed as a childcare provider and are unsure of your role in emergencies, talk with your employer to be sure you know your specific responsibilities.

In addition to employed childcare providers, parents and guardians also have a legal responsibility to give first aid to children in their care. This is called a preexisting relationship and involves a legal responsibility. A preexisting relationship also includes adults overseeing children in any situation, such as an adult who is transporting children in a vehicle or watching them at a playground.

As noted before, once you begin giving first aid, in any situation, you are obligated to continue giving care until emergency medical help takes over, another trained rescuer takes over, or you become physically exhausted.

Good Samaritan Laws

Most states have laws called **Good Samaritan laws** designed to encourage people to help others in an emergency without worrying about being sued. These laws protect adults who give first aid to other adults or children in their care, except for those employed in childcare. It is unlikely you would be found liable or financially responsible for a child's injury as long as you follow the guidelines described in this book. Ask your instructor about the specific Good Samaritan laws in your area.

Get Consent

You must have permission in order to give first aid. If you are employed at a childcare center, the center should already have the parents' permission to give emergency and other first aid to their children.

If you are the responsible adult supervising children in any other setting, and the child's parents or guardians are not present when a child is injured or becomes ill, you are assumed to have the parent's or guardian's permission to give emergency care. In a nonemergency situation you should try to reach a parent or guardian to get his or her permission, but in an emergency consent is assumed. This is called **implied consent.**

You may also encounter emergencies with adult victims of injury or sudden illness. A responsive (awake and alert) victim must give permission before you can give first aid. Tell the person you have been trained and describe what you will do to help. The victim may give permission by telling you it is okay or by nodding agreement. An unresponsive victim, however, is assumed to give consent for your help. Again, this is called implied consent.

Follow Standards of Care

Legally, you may be liable for the results of your actions if you do not follow accepted standards of care. **Standard of care** refers to what others with your same training would do in a similar situation. It is important that when you give first aid, act only as you are trained to act. Any other actions could result in the injury or illness becoming worse.

You may be guilty of **negligence** if:

1. You have a duty to act (as a childcare provider, parent or guardian, or adult with a preexisting relationship with a child).
2. You breach that duty (by not acting, or acting incorrectly).
3. Your actions or inaction causes injury or damages (including such things as physical injury or pain).

Examples of negligent actions could include moving a victim unnecessarily, doing something you have not been trained to do, or failing to give first aid as you have been trained.

Remember, once you begin giving first aid, do not stop until another trained person takes over. Stay with the victim until help arrives. If you leave the victim and the injury or illness becomes worse, this is called **abandonment.** Note that abandonment is different from justified instances of stopping care, such as if you are exhausted and unable to continue or you are in imminent danger because of hazards at the scene.

Documentation

A final legal responsibility in some childcare situations is documenting the child's injury or illness and the care you gave. Some states require such documentation. In California, for example, a special form must be filled out anytime a child receives professional medical care (including EMS personnel) while in a licensed childcare home or facility. Check with your employer about any state or facility policies for documentation.

Even if not legally required, it is a good idea whenever caring for children not your own to write down what happened and what you did. This information may be important for the child's parents or guardians and for healthcare providers who later treat the child.

COPING WITH A TRAUMATIC EVENT

Emergencies are stressful, especially with injured or ill children. When a child is seriously injured or does not survive, the incident can be traumatic for caregivers. It is important to realize that not even medical professionals can save every victim. Some injuries, illness, or circumstances are often beyond our control. If you experience such an emergency, you may have a strong reaction, or later on you may have problems coping. This is normal—we are only human, after all. To help cope with the effects of a traumatic event:

- Talk to others: family members, co-workers, local emergency responders, or your family healthcare provider (without breaching confidentiality of the victim).
- Remind yourself your reaction is normal.
- Do not be afraid or reluctant to ask for professional help. If you have an Employee Assistance Program or Member Assistance Program, they often can provide such help. Ask your personal healthcare provider who you can talk to for help.

1 Take Action in an Emergency

This chapter describes actions to take in all emergencies involving injury or illness. Always follow these basic steps:

1. Recognize the emergency and check the scene.
2. Decide to help.
3. Call 9-1-1 (when appropriate).
4. Check the injured or ill child.
5. Give first aid.
6. Ensure that the injured or ill child sees a healthcare provider (when appropriate).

Later chapters describe the specific first aid to give in different situations. This chapter describes the six steps above, how to protect yourself from infectious disease when giving first aid, and how to assess an injured or ill child.

WHAT YOU CAN DO

In any emergency, try to stay calm and confident. Remember your training. Acting calmly and confidently will help calm the injured or ill child as well.

In a childcare situation, in which other children and adults are likely to be present, consider the complete situation and others involved. While it is important to care for the injured or ill child in your care, it is also important to properly handle others who may be affected by the incident. Calm and reassure parents during an emergency with their child. Tell the parent(s) that you are trained to handle the emergency situation and what you are doing to help their child. Calm and reassure other children as well. Whenever possible, have another childcare provider supervise the other children while you provide care for the ill or injured child. Explain that you will talk with the children about what happened as soon as possible and answer their questions.

Follow these six steps in any emergency:

Recognize the Emergency and Check the Scene

You usually know there is an emergency when you see one. You see an injured or ill child, or a child acting strangely. Or you may not see a victim at first but see signs that an emergency has occurred and that someone may be hurt.

Although most childcare situations do not involve hazards to yourself and others, such hazards may be present. Always check the scene when you recognize an emergency has occurred—before rushing in to help the victim. This is particularly important when outdoors or in unfamiliar settings. You must be safe yourself if you are to help another. Look for any hazards such as the following:

- Smoke, flames
- Spilled chemicals, vapors
- Downed electrical wires
- Risk of explosion, building collapse
- Roadside dangers, high-speed traffic
- Potential personal violence

If the scene is dangerous, *stay away and call for help.* Do not become a victim yourself!

As part of checking the scene, look to see if other children are injured or ill. More help may be needed for multiple victims. Check that all children are present and make sure you are not overlooking other injuries. Look also for any clues that may help you determine what happened and what first aid may be needed. As well, look for other adults who may be able to help give first aid or go to a telephone to call 9-1-1.

Decide to Help

When you see an injured child and have determined the scene is safe, you need to act. This is not always easy. Although you may be worried about not doing the right thing, remember that you have first aid training. Once you call for help, medical professionals will be there very soon. Your goal is to help the victim until they take over.

Call 9-1-1

Call 9-1-1 (or your local emergency number) immediately if you recognize a life-threatening injury or illness. A life-threatening emergency is one in which a problem threatens the child's airway, breathing, or circulation of blood, as described later in this chapter. Do not try to transport a child to the emergency department yourself in such cases. Movement may worsen the child's condition, or the child may suddenly need additional care on the way.

If you are not sure whether a situation is serious enough to call, don't hesitate—call 9-1-1. It is better to be safe than sorry (**Figure 1-1**).

If the child is responsive and may not be seriously injured or ill, go on to the next step to check the child before calling 9-1-1—and then call 9-1-1 if needed.

Always call 9-1-1 when:

- The child may have a life-threatening condition.
- The child is unresponsive.
- The child's condition may become life threatening.
- Moving the child could make the condition worse.

Later chapters on first aid describe when to call 9-1-1 for other specific problems.

In addition to calling 9-1-1 for injury or illness, call in these situations:

- Fire, explosion
- Vehicle crash
- Downed electrical wire
- Chemical spill, gas leak, or the presence of any unknown substances

How to Call EMS

When you call 9-1-1 or your local emergency number, be ready to give the following information:

- Your name and the phone number you are using
- The location and number of injured or ill children—specific enough for the arriving crew to find them
- What happened to the child and any special circumstances or conditions that may require special rescue or medical equipment
- The child's condition: For example, is the child responsive? Breathing? Bleeding?
- The child's approximate age and sex
- What is being done for the child

It is important to not hang up until the dispatcher instructs you to, because you may be given advice on how to care for the child.

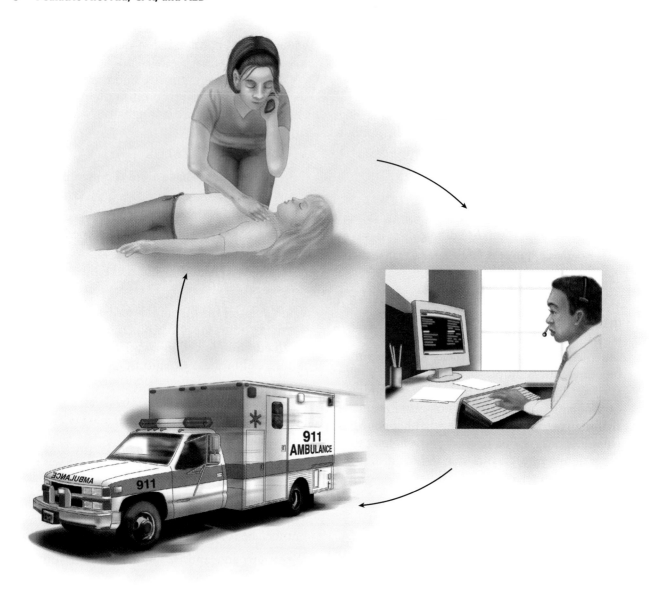

Figure 1-1 Call 9-1-1.

If other adults are present, ask them to call 9-1-1 while you go on to check the child and give first aid.

Check the Victim

First check the child and care for life-threatening conditions requiring immediate first aid.

Give First Aid

Give first aid once you have checked the child and know his or her condition. Later chapters give the first aid steps for the conditions you are likely to find. In many cases first aid involves simple actions you can take to help the victim.

Get the Victim to a Healthcare Provider

You may have decided at first that the child's condition was not an emergency and did not call 9-1-1. In many cases, however, the child still needs to see a healthcare provider. If you have any doubt, call 9-1-1. If you are employed in a childcare center, follow your center's policy regarding contacting the child's parents. Later chapters on specific conditions requiring first aid describe when a victim needs to go to the emergency department or see a healthcare provider.

AVOIDING INFECTION

In any emergency situation there is some risk of a first aider getting an infectious disease from a victim who has a disease. That risk is very low, however, and taking steps to prevent being infected greatly reduces that risk. You can take precautions to prevent transmission of bloodborne and airborne infectious diseases.

Bloodborne Disease

Several serious diseases can be transmitted from one person to another through contact with the infected person's blood. These are called bloodborne diseases. Bacteria or viruses that cause such diseases, called pathogens, are also present in some other body fluids, such as semen, vaginal secretions, and bloody saliva or vomit. Other body fluids, such as nasal secretions, sweat, tears, and urine, do not normally transmit pathogens. Three serious bloodborne infections are HIV, hepatitis B, and hepatitis C.

HIV

The human immunodeficiency virus (HIV) is the pathogen that eventually causes AIDS (acquired immunodeficiency syndrome). AIDS is a fatal disease transmitted from one person to another only through body fluids.

Because HIV can be transmitted through pregnancy and occasionally through breast milk, some children in childcare situations may have the virus. There have been no known cases, however, of the virus spreading from one child to another in childcare settings or schools. Nonetheless, childcare providers should always take precautions when blood or body fluids of *any* child or adult victim are involved (see following sections).

Note that a child's medical record is confidential. If you are employed in a childcare center, follow your center's policies when caring for a child known to have HIV.

Remember that HIV is transmitted only through certain body fluids. It is not spread through regular daily activities such as touching, coughing or sneezing, sharing foods, sharing a restroom, or playing together.

Hepatitis B

Hepatitis B (HBV) is a viral infectious disease of the liver transmitted through contact with an infected person's body fluids. The disease is difficult to treat and often remains in the person for life, possibly leading to liver damage or cancer.

A vaccine is available for HBV. Individuals who are more likely to come in contact with HBV-infected people, such as healthcare workers and professional rescuers, often get this vaccine. The law requires that such employees who are at risk for HBV exposure be offered free vaccinations by their employer.

Hepatitis C

Hepatitis C (HCV) is another bloodborne viral disease that can cause liver disease or cancer. It cannot be cured, and there is no vaccine. Following the same precautions to protect against transmission of HIV will also prevent transmission of HBV and HCV.

WEST NILE VIRUS

West Nile virus (WNV) is a relatively new bloodborne disease now established as a seasonal epidemic in parts of North America. Less than 1% of people infected with WNV develop severe illness, however, and about 80% have no signs and symptoms at all. WNV is spread mostly by the bite of infected mosquitoes. The best way to avoid WNV is to prevent mosquito bites with personal protection, such as wearing long sleeves and pants and reducing mosquito breeding sites.

Protection Against Bloodborne Disease

Because these bloodborne diseases cannot be cured, they should be prevented. The best prevention is to avoid contact with *all* victims' blood and body fluids. You cannot know whether a child or other victim (even a close friend) may be infected, because often these diseases do not produce signs and symptoms. Even the victim may not know that he or she is infected.

The Centers for Disease Control and Prevention (CDC) therefore recommends taking **universal precautions** whenever giving first aid. *Universal* means for all victims, all the time. Always assume that blood and body fluids may be infected. Use the following recommended precautions to prevent coming into contact with a victim's blood or body fluids:

- Use personal protective equipment.
- If you do not have medical exam gloves with you, put your hands in plastic bags or use another barrier between you and the blood or body fluid.
- Wash your hands with soap and water before and after giving first aid.
- Cover any cuts or scrapes in your skin with protective clothing or gloves.
- Do not touch your mouth, nose, or eyes when giving first aid (e.g., do not eat, drink, or smoke).
- Do not touch objects soiled with blood or body fluids.
- Be careful to avoid being cut by anything sharp at the emergency scene, such as broken glass or torn metal.
- Use absorbent material to soak up spilled blood or body fluids, and dispose of appropriately; clean the area with a commercial disinfectant or a freshly made 10% bleach solution.
- If you are exposed to a victim's blood or body fluid, wash immediately with soap and water and call your healthcare provider. At work, report the situation to your supervisor.

See also Chapter 14 on preventing illness in child-care settings.

Personal Protective Equipment

Personal protective equipment (PPE) is any equipment used to protect yourself from contact with blood or other body fluids. Most important, keep medical exam gloves in your first aid kit and wear them in most first aid situations (**Figure 1-2**).

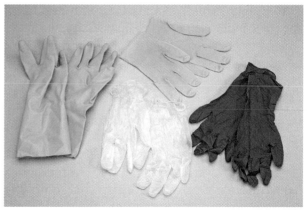

Figure 1-2. Wear gloves to protect yourself from contact with blood or other body fluids.

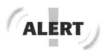

ALERT

Latex Gloves

Medical exam gloves are often made of latex rubber, to which some people are allergic. Signs and symptoms of latex allergy may include skin rashes, hives, itching skin or eyes, flushing, watering or swollen eyes, a runny nose, or an asthmatic reaction. Use gloves made of vinyl or other material if you have any of these symptoms or if you know the victim has a latex allergy.

A pocket face mask or face shield is a barrier device used when giving CPR. This device should be in the first aid kit, and you should always use it for added protection. Because giving CPR with a barrier device can greatly reduce the chance of an infectious disease being transmitted from or to a victim, barrier devices are always recommended (**Figure 1-3**).

Airborne Disease

Infectious diseases may also be transmitted through the air, especially from a victim who is coughing or sneezing. Tuberculosis (TB) has made a comeback in the last decade and is sometimes resistant to treatment.

Healthcare workers use precautions when caring for people known or suspected to have TB, but rarely does a first aider need to take special precautions against airborne disease.

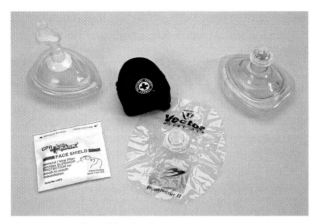

Figure 1-3. Variety of barrier devices.

In 2003 an outbreak of severe acute respiratory syndrome (SARS) in some parts of the world caused a new scare. SARS is primarily an airborne infectious disease, transmitted when an infected person coughs or sneezes within close proximity to others. During the 2003 epidemic almost 10% of the approximately 8,000 known SARS victims in the world died. Only 7 people in the United States were known to have contracted SARS, all through international travel to epidemic areas. The CDC continues to monitor the risks of SARS and will issue updates and warnings if new outbreaks occur.

First aiders who want to learn more about preventing bloodborne and airborne disease are encouraged to take the National Safety Council course on Bloodborne and Airborne Pathogens.

CHECK THE INJURED OR ILL CHILD

As described earlier, after you recognize the emergency, check the scene for safety, and call 9-1-1 if appropriate, you then check the child to see what problems may need first aid. This check, called an **assessment,** has three steps:

1. Check for immediate life-threatening conditions.
2. Get the victim's history (find out what happened and what may have contributed to the emergency).
3. Check the rest of the child's body (perform a physical examination).

While giving first aid and waiting for help to arrive, continue with a fourth step:

4. Monitor the child for any changes.

Always perform these steps in this order. If there is an immediate life-threatening problem, such as stopped breathing, the child needs immediate help. This victim could die if you first spent time looking for broken bones or asking bystanders what happened. *Always remember:* Check first for breathing and severe bleeding.

Check for Life-Threatening Problems

In less than a minute you can check the child for immediate life-threatening conditions. This involves checking for:

- Unresponsiveness
- Lack of breathing
- Severe bleeding

Unless the child is obviously alert, **check for responsiveness.** Tap the child on the shoulder and ask if he or she is okay, or flick the heels of an infant. A child is responsive if he or she speaks to you, moves purposefully, or otherwise responds to stimuli. A child who does not respond is called unresponsive. An unresponsive child is considered to have a potentially life-threatening condition. Immediately call for help so that someone calls 9-1-1. If the victim is unresponsive, continue checking for problems.

After checking for responsiveness, check next for the presence or absence of breathing. **A child who can speak or cough is breathing.** In an unresponsive child, to check breathing, you must ensure that the airway is open. The airway is the route air takes from the mouth and nose through the throat and down to the lungs. The airway may be blocked by something stuck in the throat, by swollen tissue, or by an unresponsive child's own tongue.

In an unresponsive child, you may need to open the airway. If the child is lying on the back, face up, you must prevent the tongue from obstructing the airway by positioning the child's head to open the airway. This is done by tilting the head back and lifting the chin as shown in

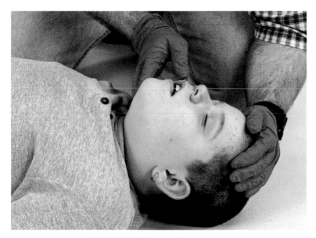

Figure 1-4 Head tilt–chin lift.

Figure 1-4. This is called the head tilt–chin lift. This position moves the tongue away from the opening into the throat to allow air to pass through the airway.

With the airway open, check for breathing. Lean over with your ear close to the child's mouth and nose, and **look** at the child's chest to see if it rises and falls with breathing. **Listen** for any sounds of breathing, and **feel** for breath on your cheek. If you do not detect breathing within 10 seconds, assume the child is not breathing. Lack of breathing may be caused by an obstructed airway (choking) or other causes. If the child is not breathing, you must immediately start CPR as described in the next chapter.

After ensuring that the child is breathing, next check for severe bleeding. If the child is bleeding profusely, vital organs are not receiving enough oxygen to sustain life. Check for severe bleeding by quickly looking over the child's body for obvious blood. Check for blood-saturated clothing or blood pooled under the body. Control any severe bleeding with direct pressure (see Chapter 3).

This step completes the initial assessment (see Perform the Skill: Initial Assessment).

Get a History

If you find no immediate life-threatening conditions you must care for, continue to check the child for other problems and try to find out more about what happened. Ask the child simple questions, such as "What happened?" and "Where does it hurt?" Ask other people about what they know or saw.

It is important to try to get information about the child and the problem, called "the history," to help you decide what first aid to give. This information is also important for healthcare providers who may later treat the child. Use the **SAMPLE** history format:

S = ***Signs and symptoms.*** What can you observe about the child's problem (**signs**)? Ask the child how he or she feels (**symptoms**).

A = ***Allergies.*** Ask an older child or a parent about any allergies to foods, medicines, insect stings, or other substances. Look for a medical ID bracelet. In a childcare setting, someone can check the child's file for such information (**Figure 1-5**).

M = ***Medications.*** Find out if the child is taking any prescribed medications or over-the-counter products.

P = ***Previous problems.*** Find out if the child has had a problem like this before or has any other illnesses.

L = ***Last food or drink.*** Find out what and when the child last ate or drank.

E = ***Events.*** Ask the child and others what happened, and try to identify the events that led to the current situation.

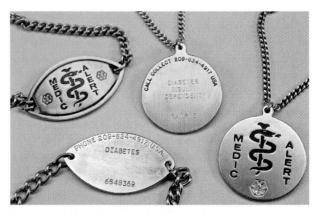

Figure 1-5. Examples of medical ID jewelry.

Perform the Skill

Initial Assessment

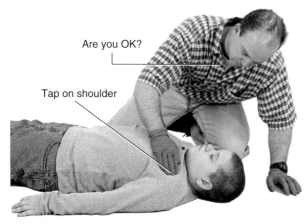

Are you OK?

Tap on shoulder

1 Check responsiveness.

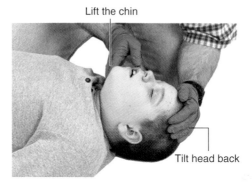

Lift the chin

Tilt head back

2 Open the airway.

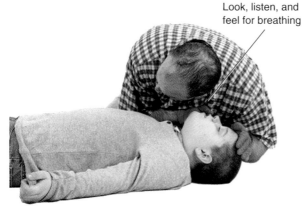

Look, listen, and feel for breathing

3 Check for breathing.

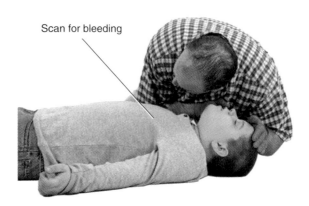

Scan for bleeding

4 Check for severe bleeding.

Physical Examination

The third step of the assessment of an injured or ill child is the physical examination. With this examination you may find other injuries that need first aid or additional clues to a child's condition. It is important to note, however, that you do not stop giving first aid for a serious condition just to do this examination. Instead, keep the child still and calm and wait for EMS professionals.

The physical examination includes examining the child from toe to head looking for anything out of the ordinary. Starting at the toes and working up to the head allows a child to get used to you in a more nonthreatening manner. As a general rule look for the following signs and symptoms of injury or illness throughout the body:

- Pain when an area is touched
- Bleeding or wounds
- An area that is swollen or deformed from its usual appearance

- Skin color (flushed or pale), temperature (hot or cold), moisture (dry, sweating, clammy)
- Abnormal sensation or movement of the area

Monitor the Child

Give first aid for injuries or illness you discover as you assess the child. With very minor conditions the child may need no more than your first aid. In other situations the child may need to see a healthcare provider or go to an emergency department. With all life-threatening or serious conditions, you should have had someone call 9-1-1, and you are now awaiting the arrival of help.

While waiting for help, stay with the child and make sure his or her condition does not worsen. With an unresponsive child or a victim with a serious injury, check for breathing at least every 5 minutes.

MOVING A CHILD

Never move a seriously injured or ill child unless you have to for his or her own safety. Movement can worsen the condition. Wait for the arriving crew to move the child with their appropriate equipment and training.

If the scene is unsafe, you may need to move an injured or ill child. For example, you may need to remove a child from the risk of fire or poisoning by toxic fumes or substances. If the child is not suspected to have a spinal injury and is not too heavy, you can carry the child away from the danger. Lift with your legs rather than your back, and hold the child close to your body for support.

If you think the child may have a spinal injury, you must support the head and neck in line with the body when moving the child. One way to do this, if you are alone, is with the shoulder or clothes drag, using your forearms to support the child's head while pulling him or her away from the danger (**Figure 1-6**).

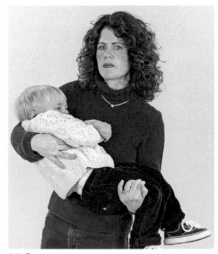
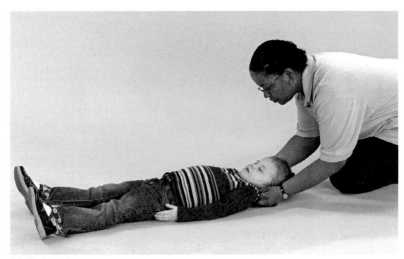

(a) One-person carry   (b) Clothes drag

Figure 1-6 Emergency moves for children.

Perform the Skill

Physical Examination of Injured Child

Feel each leg from toes to thighs for sensation, pain, deformity, and bleeding. Check feet for signs of circulation

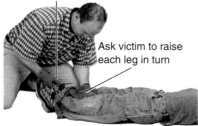

Ask victim to raise each leg in turn

1 Check lower extremities.

Check from fingers to shoulders for sensation, pain, deformity, and bleeding

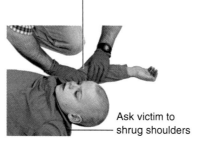

Ask victim to shrug shoulders

2 Check upper extremities. Look for medical ID bracelet.

Gently sqeeze pelvis to detect pain or deformity

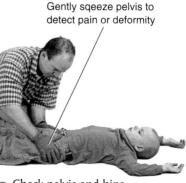

3 Check pelvis and hips.

Gently check for rigidity, pain, or bleeding

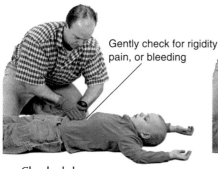

4 Check abdomen.

Check for movement of breathing, pain, deformity, and wounds

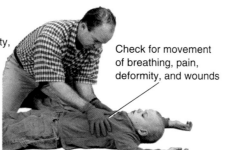

5 Check chest. Ask victim to breathe deeply.

6 Check skin appearance, temperature, moisture.

Do not move the neck

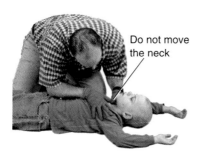

7 Check neck area for medical ID necklace, deformity or swelling, and pain.

Check pupils: equal size, react to light

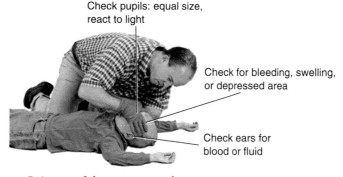

Check for bleeding, swelling, or depressed area

Check ears for blood or fluid

8 Being careful not to move the child's head or neck, check the head. If you find any problems in any body area, do not let the victim move. Wait for help to arrive.

Chapter

2 Basic Life Support

Basic life support (BLS) refers to first aid given if the victim's breathing or heart stops. Many things can cause breathing or the heart to stop. BLS is often needed for victims of:

- Heart problems

- Drowning

- Choking

- Other injuries or conditions that affect breathing or the heart

If a child's heart stops beating, breathing will stop too. If breathing stops first for any reason, the heart will stop also. The child will need cardiopulmonary resuscitation (CPR). CPR is also used for a choking victim who becomes unresponsive.

OVERVIEW OF BLS

Giving BLS involves one or more lifesaving skills, depending on the child's needs. These skills are sometimes called **resuscitation** and include:

- *Rescue breaths* to get needed oxygen into the lungs
- *Chest compressions* to pump oxygenated blood to vital organs
- Use of an *automated external defibrillator (AED)* to shock the heart to beat regularly
- *Choking care,* including chest compressions, to expel an obstructing object from the airway

Pediatric Differences

Because of size and other differences, some BLS skills are used somewhat differently in children and infants than in adults. The exact technique to use depends on the child's age. Standard age groups are defined in the following way:

Infant — birth to 1 year

Child — ages 1 to 8

Adult — over age 8

The chart at the end of this chapter summarizes the differences in techniques among adults, children, and infants.

Cardiac Chain of Survival

BLS includes care given to any victim whose breathing or circulation stops. Circulation stops when the heart stops beating, a condition called **cardiac arrest.** In adults, the most common cause of sudden cardiac arrest is heart attack. Fortunately, heart attack and

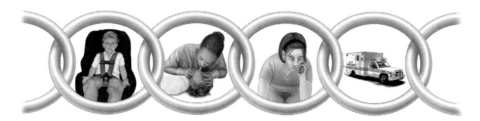

Figure 2-1 Pediatric chain of survival.

other heart problems are very rare in children, although other causes of cardiac arrest, such as choking, are more common in children than in adults. Causes of sudden cardiac arrest in children include:

- Choking (if breathing is not restored quickly)
- Drowning
- Poisoning
- Electrocution
- Traumatic injury
- Heart problems

To recognize the urgent need for quick action to save the life of someone whose heart has stopped, the Citizen CPR Foundation created the concept of the pediatric **chain of survival.** This chain has four crucial links (**Figure 2-1**):

1. **Prevention of injuries and cardiac arrest.** Take steps to prevent the many causes of injury and sudden cardiac arrest in children.
2. **Early bystander CPR.** For an unresponsive child who is not breathing, start CPR immediately.
3. **Early access to EMS.** Call, or have someone call, to get help on the way. Send someone right away to get an AED for children age 1 and older.
4. **Early pediatric advanced life support.** The sooner the victim is treated by emergency care professionals, the better the chance for survival. You can help make sure the victim reaches this last link in the chain by acting immediately.

THE RECOVERY POSITION

An unresponsive child without a suspected spinal injury who is breathing when found or after receiving BLS should be put in the recovery position. This position:

- Helps keep the airway open
- Allows fluids to drain from the mouth
- Prevents inhaling stomach contents if the child vomits

Once the child is in the recovery position, continue to monitor the child's breathing (**Figure 2-2**).

BLS FOR CHILDREN

The following BLS techniques—rescue breaths, CPR, use of an AED, and choking care—are described for children from 1 to 8 years of age. Remember to vary your technique appropriately for older children (over age 8 considered an adult).

Call First/Call Fast

With any unresponsive victim, if someone else is present at the scene, have that person call 9-1-1 immediately. Shout for anyone who may hear you, and have them call 9-1-1 and go for an AED.

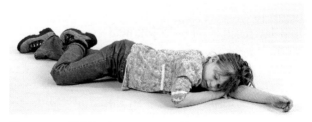

Figure 2-2 Child in the recovery position.

Perform the Skill

Recovery Position

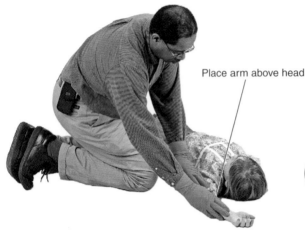

Place arm above head

1 Position the child's arm.

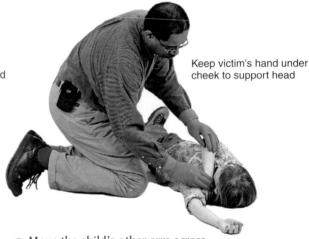

Keep victim's hand under cheek to support head

2 Move the child's other arm across chest and against cheek.

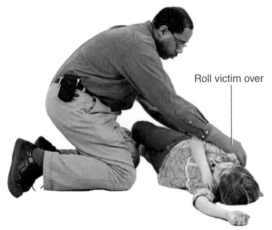

Roll victim over

3 Bend the child's leg and roll the child onto his or her side.

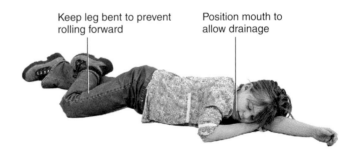

Keep leg bent to prevent rolling forward

Position mouth to allow drainage

4 Adjust the child's position as needed to ensure the airway remains open.

When you are alone, however, you need to decide whether to call immediately or to first begin to provide care for the victim. The rule that lay rescuers should follow depends on the victim's age. An infant or child who is found unresponsive is likely to be experiencing an airway or breathing problem and less likely to need defibrillation. For an infant or child, therefore, if you are alone with the victim and no one hears your shouts for help, you should give 5 cycles of chest compressions and rescue breaths (about 2 minutes of CPR) before pausing to call 9-1-1 and then continuing to provide CPR. **Remember: For an infant or child, start CPR first, but call fast.**

An adult who is found unresponsive, however, is more likely to be the victim of a heart attack and therefore needs defibrillation urgently. For an adult, therefore, if you are alone with the victim, call 9-1-1 immediately and then return to provide CPR. **Remember: Call first, for an adult.**

RESCUE BREATHS

Giving rescue breaths is a technique of blowing air into a nonbreathing child's lungs to oxygenate the blood. Rescue breaths are given along with chest compressions, which help circulate the oxygenated blood to vital organs, keeping the child alive until the child is resuscitated or EMS personnel arrive to give advanced care.

Rescue breaths are given along with chest compressions to any child who is not breathing. Give two rescue breaths immediately when you discover the child is not breathing. Then begin CPR. Have someone call 9-1-1 immediately. If an AED is available, send someone to get it.

Techniques for Giving Rescue Breaths

First position the child on his or her back. Open the airway using the head tilt–chin lift. Use a barrier device to protect against disease transmission if you have one, but do not delay giving rescue breaths to get one. Even without a barrier device the risk of contracting an infectious disease from providing rescue breaths is very low.

The basic technique is to blow air into the child while watching the chest rise to make sure your air is going into the lungs. Do not try to rush the air in or blow too forcefully. Do not take a big breath in order to exhale more air into the child; just take a normal breath as usual. Give each breath over about 1 second. If the breath does not go in, or if you feel resistance or do not see the child's chest rise, try again to open the airway and give two breaths. Then start chest compressions. Remember these key points:

- Do not blow harder than is needed to make the child's chest rise.
- After each breath remember to let the air escape and the chest fall.
- Blowing in too forcefully or for too long is ineffective and may put air in the stomach, which may cause vomiting.

Mouth-to-Barrier

Barrier devices are always recommended when giving rescue breaths. Position a pocket mask or face shield on the child's face and give breaths through the device. Make sure it is sealed to the child's face. Make sure your air is going into the child by watching the chest rise. When using a face shield, pinch the child's nose closed when giving a breath (**Figure 2-3**).

Mouth-to-Mouth

If you do not have a barrier device, pinch the child's nose shut and seal your mouth over the child's mouth. Breathe into the child's mouth, watching the chest rise to confirm the air going in.

Mouth-to-Nose

Give rescue breaths through the child's nose if the mouth cannot be opened or is injured, or if you cannot get a good seal with your mouth over the child's. Hold the child's mouth closed, seal your mouth over the nose and give a breath, then let the mouth open to let the air escape.

Mouth-to-Stoma

Because of past illness or injury, some children breathe through a hole in their lower neck called a stoma. Check this hole to see if the child is breathing. If the child is not breathing, cup your hand over the victim's nose and mouth, seal your barrier device (or your mouth) over the stoma, and give rescue breaths as usual (**Figure 2-4**).

Rescue Breaths for Infants

Rescue breaths for infants are similar to those for children, with these differences:

- Gently tilt the head back to open the airway and check for breathing—do not overextend the neck.
- Cover both the mouth and the nose with your mouth to give breaths (use the mouth or nose only if you cannot cover both).
- Give breaths in shallow puffs of air lasting 1 second each.

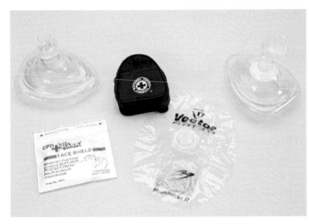

(a) Barrier devices

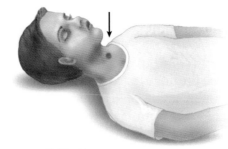

Figure 2-4 Child with a stoma.

CARDIOPULMONARY RESUSCITATION (CPR)

About 4 minutes after the heart stops beating, brain damage begins to occur. The more time that passes without resuscitation, the less likely it is that CPR will be successful. It is crucial to quickly recognize the need for CPR and start it immediately in a child whose heart has stopped.

CPR combines rescue breaths (to get oxygen into the victim's lungs) with chest compressions (to pump the oxygenated blood to vital organs). Give CPR to any victim who is not breathing. CPR is also used for an unresponsive choking victim because the chest compressions can expel a foreign object from the victim's airway.

Technique of CPR

The general technique of CPR involves alternating chest compressions and rescue breaths. After checking the victim and determining the absence of breathing, start chest compressions immediately after giving the initial 2 rescue breaths. For a victim of any age, these are the general steps of CPR:

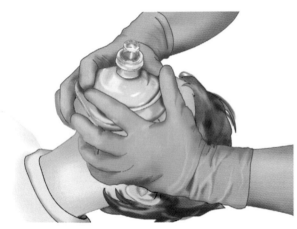

(b) Position pocket mask over mouth and nose

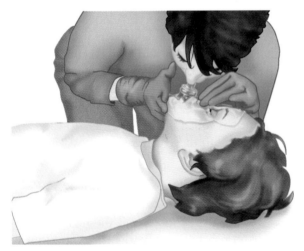

(c) Position barrier device over mouth and pinch nose

Figure 2-3 Mouth-to-barrier rescue breathing.

1. Find the correct hand position on the lower half of the breastbone midway between the nipples in adults and children, or just below this line in infants, as shown in **Figure 2-5**. For adults, place the heel of one hand in the correct position; then put the second hand on top of the first and interlock fingers. For children, depending on their size and your strength, use both hands or the heel of one hand. For infants, use two fingers.

2. Compress the chest hard and fast at a rate of 100 compressions per minute.

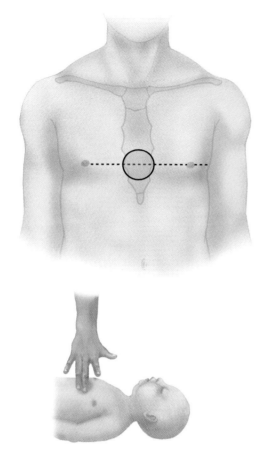

Figure 2-5 Proper hand placement for chest compressions on a child or an adult (top) and an infant (bottom).

Note that this is the *rate, or speed, for giving compressions*—not the number of compressions actually given—since it is necessary to stop compressions to give rescue breaths. Compressions in an adult should be 1½ to 2 inches deep. In an infant or child, compressions should be one-third to one-half the depth of the chest. Release completely between compressions to let the chest return to its normal height, but do not take your hands or fingers from the chest.

3. Alternate 30 chest compressions and 2 rescue breaths. Give each breath for 1 second.

Compression-Only CPR

An unresponsive, nonbreathing child needs both rescue breaths and chest compressions to move oxygenated blood to vital organs.

However, if for any reason you cannot or will not give rescue breaths, still give the child chest compressions. This gives the child a better chance for survival than doing nothing.

AUTOMATED EXTERNAL DEFIBRILLATORS (AEDs)

Not every child who receives BLS needs an AED, but some do. Remember the chain of survival. An AED should be used with a child who is not breathing. In cases of cardiac arrest the AED may restart a normal heartbeat.

Pediatric AED pads are available in some facilities for use by trained rescuers and first aiders. Use pediatric AED pads for a child under age 8 or 55 lbs, if available. If not, use adult AED pads. In most areas a healthcare provider oversees placement and use of the AED, and your AED training must meet certain requirements. For professional rescuers, this is called **medical direction.** Your course instructor will inform you how to meet the legal requirements in your area for using an AED.

How AEDs Work

The heart functions to pump blood to the lungs to pick up oxygen and then pump oxygenated blood to all parts of the body. The heart consists of four chambers—the left atrium, the right atrium, and the left and right ventricles. The ventricles, the lower chambers of the heart, do most of the pumping. The heart's electrical system keeps the four chambers of the heart synchronized and working together. The sinus and atrioventricular (AV) nodes help organize and control the rhythmic electrical impulses that keep the heart beating properly (**Figure 2-6**).

In some situations involving trauma, electrocution, drowning, poisoning, congenital heart disease, or other causes, the electrical system of a child's heart may be disrupted, causing an abnormal heart rhythm.

Ventricular fibrillation (V-fib) is an abnormal heart rhythm that stops circulation of the blood. Although we say a victim in V-fib is in cardiac arrest, the heart is not actually completely still but is beating abnormally. **Fibrillation** means

Perform the Skill

CPR

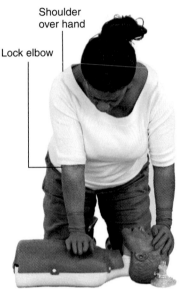

Shoulder over hand

Lock elbow

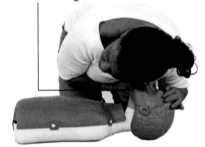

Look, listen, and feel for breathing

1 Open the airway and determine if the victim is not breathing.

2 Give 2 rescue breaths, each lasting 1 second, that make the chest rise. (If the first breath does not go in, reposition the head and try again.)

3 Put hand(s) in correct position for chest compressions.

4 Give 30 chest compressions at rate of 100 per minute. Count aloud for a steady fast rate: "One, two, three, . . . " Then give 2 breaths.

5 Continue cycles of 30 compressions and 2 breaths.

6 Continue CPR until:
• The victim begins to move,
   • an AED is brought to the scene and is ready to use,
   • professional help arrives and takes over, or
   • you are too exhausted to continue.

7 a. If the victim starts moving, check for breathing. If the victim is breathing and no spinal injury is suspected, put the victim in the recovery position and monitor breathing.
   b. When an AED arrives, start the AED sequence.

ALERT

Chest Compressions

• Be careful with your hand position for chest compressions. Keep fingers off the chest.
• Do not give compressions over the bottom tip of the breastbone.
• When compressing, keep your elbows straight and keep your hands in contact with the chest at all times.
• Remember to compress the chest hard and fast, but let the chest recoil completely between compressions.
• Minimize the amount of time used giving rescue breaths between sets of compressions.

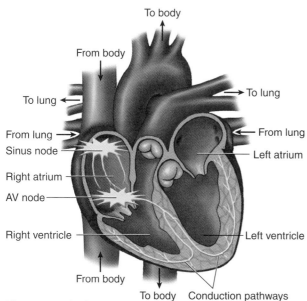

Figure 2-6 The heart.

the ventricles of the heart are quivering instead of beating rhythmically. Blood is not filling the ventricles and is not being pumped out to the lungs or body as normal.

The AED automatically checks the child's heart rhythm and advises whether the child needs a shock. If the victim's heart is in V-fib, the unit will advise giving an electric shock to return the heart to a normal rhythm. This is called **defibrillation,** or stopping the fibrillation of the heart.

Current AEDs are easy and simple to use, but they must be used right away. With every minute that goes by before defibrillation begins, the child's chances for survival drop by about 10%.

The AED

AEDs are complex inside but simple to use. They contain a battery and are portable. The unit has two pads connected to it with cables. These pads are placed on the child's body. The unit then analyzes the victim's heart rhythm and advises whether to give a shock. Some models have a screen that tells you what to do; all models give directions in a clear voice. Different AED models vary somewhat in other features, but all work in the same basic way. AEDs for use on children have special pediatric pads that are clearly labeled for use on children (**Figure 2-7**).

Using an AED

In any situation in which a child suddenly collapses or is found unresponsive, be thinking about the possibility of cardiac arrest even as you come up to the child. If someone else is present and you know an AED is available, send that person to get it *now*. It's better to have it right away and not use it than to need it and have to wait for it.

Determine the Need for an AED

As always, first check the child's breathing. If the child is unresponsive and not breathing, send someone to call 9-1-1 and to get an AED.

Start CPR

Remember the BLS steps and the chain of survival. Give CPR until the AED arrives at the scene and is ready to use. If you arrive at the scene of a sudden witnessed cardiac arrest with the AED, use the AED immediately before starting CPR. An easy way to remember when to use an AED is that if you need to perform CPR on a victim, then you should also apply an AED if available.

Attach the AED

Be sure the child is not in water or in contact with metal. Water or metal conduct electricity that may pose a risk to you or others. Place the AED beside the child, turn it on, and attach

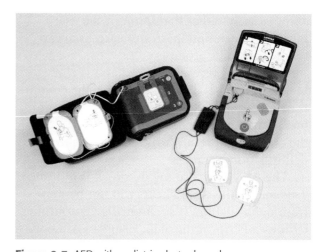

Figure 2-7 AED with pediatric electrode pads.

the pads (electrodes) on the child's body as illustrated on the pads.

Attach the AED pads to the child only if the child is unresponsive and not breathing. Expose the child's chest, and dry the skin with a towel or dry clothing if the skin is damp. Remove the backing from the pads and apply the pads firmly on the child's body in the positions indicated by the AED manufacturer. If required with your AED model, plug the pad cables into the main unit.

Analyze and Shock

When the pads are in place and the AED unit is on, most AED models then automatically analyze the child's heart rhythm. Do not move or touch the child while it is analyzing. After it analyzes the heart rhythm, the unit will advise you whether to give a shock or to continue CPR. If a shock is advised, be sure no one is touching the child. Look up and down the child and say, "Everybody clear!" Once everyone is clear, administer the shock (when advised). After the shock, immediately give CPR for 5 cycles of 30 compressions and 2 breaths (about 2 minutes). Then the AED will analyze again, and it will advise another shock, if needed, or continuing CPR (with the pads left in place).

Note that different AEDs may use different prompts. Follow the unit's voice and picture prompts through this process. Some units can be programmed to administer the shock automatically rather than prompt the user to push the shock button; in this case, as always, follow the unit's prompts.

If the child recovers (moves and is breathing) and is unresponsive, put the child in the recovery position and continue to monitor breathing. Keep the AED pads in place, because the child might return to V-fib and require defibrillation again.

The AED may also say no shock is indicated. This means the child's heart will not benefit from defibrillation. If so, immediately continue CPR (see Perform the Skill: Using an AED on an Infant or Child).

ALERT

AED

Do not use a cell phone or two-way radio within 6 feet of an AED.

Special Situations

Some situations involve special considerations in the use of the AED.

Infants

Currently AED use on both adults and children from age 1 to 8 is recommended. AED use for infants is not recommended against, but the evidence is considered "indeterminate" regarding the benefit of AED use for infants versus the risks of incorrectly analyzing rhythm or delivering an inappropriate shock level. There are proponents for infant AED use, however, and AED manufacturers claim AEDs are safe and appropriate when using the correct pediatric pads. Follow the guidelines you learn in your AED training and the policies of your childcare center.

Injured Victims

Cardiac arrest in a severely injured child is usually caused by the traumatic injury, not by a heart rhythm problem like V-fib. In such cases your local medical direction may specify not to use the AED. However, if the injury seems minor, the child's cardiac arrest may respond to defibrillation. You should attach the pads and follow the prompts from the AED.

Hypothermia Victims

Determining whether a victim of hypothermia (low body temperature) is breathing can be difficult. Handle a hypothermic child very carefully because jarring may cause cardiac arrest. Follow your local guidelines for AED use if the child is not breathing. Typically, if the AED finds a shockable rhythm and advises shocks, only one shock is given, and then CPR is performed

Perform the Skill

Using an AED on an Infant or Child

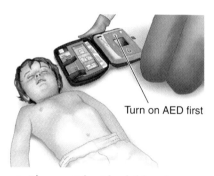

Turn on AED first

1 Position child away from water and metal.

2 Place unit beside child and turn it on.

3 Expose child's torso and dry the area if necessary.

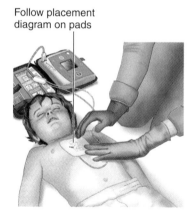

Follow placement diagram on pads

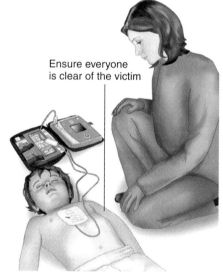

Ensure everyone is clear of the victim

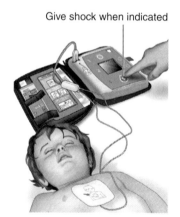

Give shock when indicated

4 Apply pads to child's torso. If needed, plug cables into unit.

5 Stay clear during rhythm analysis.

6 Follow prompts from AED unit to:
a. Press shock button or
b. Do not shock; and give CPR starting with chest compressions.

7 Stand clear when AED prompts to analyze the rhythm again after 5 cycles of CPR (about 2 minutes).

8 Continue steps 6 and 7 until the child moves or professional rescuers arrive and take over.

9 If the victim recovers (moves), check for breathing and put a breathing unresponsive victim in the recovery position (with pads remaining in place) and continue to monitor the breathing.

until help arrives. Note that many victims of hypothermia can be resuscitated even after a prolonged period of time. In this case always attempt resuscitation even if a long time has elapsed.

Potential AED Problems

An AED must be maintained regularly and the battery kept charged. With regular maintenance an AED should not have any problems during use.

The AED may also prompt you to avoid problems. If you get a low-battery prompt, change the battery before continuing. Another prompt may advise you to prevent moving the child, if the AED detects motion.

AED Maintenance

AEDs require regular maintenance. Check the manual from the manufacturer for periodic scheduled maintenance and testing of the unit. A daily inspection of the unit helps ensure the AED is always ready for use and all needed supplies are present. Professional rescuers usually inspect the unit at the beginning of their shift. Most facilities with an AED use a daily checklist form. A checklist should always be adapted for the specific AED model, including the manufacturer's daily maintenance guidelines. In addition, many units come with a simulator device to be used to check that the AED is correctly analyzing rhythms and delivering shocks; this may be part of the daily inspection routine.

CHOKING (AIRWAY OBSTRUCTION)

Choking is a total or partial obstruction of the airway. It occurs commonly in infants and small children who put objects in their mouths and in children when eating. With a total obstruction, the child becomes unresponsive within minutes. CPR is given to an unresponsive child because the chest thrusts may expel the foreign object (see Perform the Skill: Care for Choking Child).

Care for Choking

When You See

In a responsive child:
- Coughing, wheezing, difficulty breathing
- Clutching at throat
- Pale or bluish coloring around mouth and nailbeds
- Acting panicked and desperate

Do This First

1. If the child is coughing, encourage continued coughing to clear the object.
2. If not coughing, ask if the child can breathe or speak. If the child cannot, give abdominal thrusts.
3. If the child becomes unresponsive, start CPR. If alone, call 9-1-1 after 5 cycles of chest compressions and rescue breaths (about 2 minutes).

Additional Care

- Continue to give abdominal thrusts until the object comes out or the child becomes unresponsive.

Choking Infant

Choking care for infants is somewhat different from that for children. If a choking infant is crying or coughing, watch carefully to see if the object comes out. If a choking responsive infant is not crying or coughing, assume the airway is obstructed. Rather than abdominal thrusts as with a child, an infant is given alternating back slaps and chest thrusts (see Perform the Skill: Care for Choking Infant).

If a choking infant becomes unresponsive, send someone to call 9-1-1, and start CPR. Check for an object in the mouth each time before you give a breath, and remove any object you see with your fingers.

Perform the Skill

Care for Choking Child

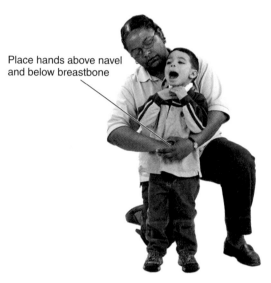

Place hands above navel
and below breastbone

1 Kneel or stand behind the child and reach around the abdomen.

2 Make a fist with one hand and grasp it with the other (thumb side into abdomen).

3 Thrust inward and upward into the abdomen with quick jerks.

4 Continue until the child can expel the object or becomes unresponsive.

5 If the child becomes unresponsive, give CPR. Look inside the mouth before giving breaths, and remove any object you see.

Perform the Skill

Care for Choking Infant

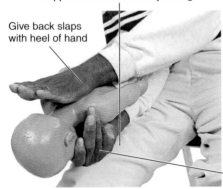

Support infant's torso on your leg

Give back slaps with heel of hand

Support infant's head and neck

1 Support the infant's head in one hand, with the torso on your forearm on your thigh. Give up to five back slaps between the shoulder blades.

2 Check for expelled object. If object not expelled, continue with next step.

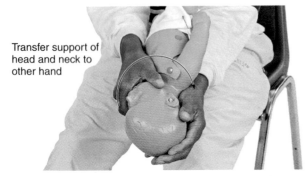

Transfer support of head and neck to other hand

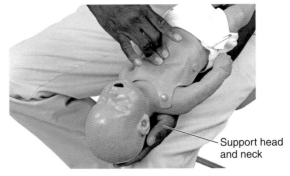

Support head and neck

3 With other hand on back of infant's head, roll the infant face up.

4 Give up to five chest thrusts with middle and ring fingers. Check mouth for expelled object.

5 Repeat steps 1 to 4, alternating back slaps and chest thrusts and checking the mouth. Continue until after object is expelled or infant becomes unresponsive.

6 If the infant becomes unresponsive, give CPR. Look inside mouth before giving breaths, and remove any object you see.

Summary of Basic Life Support

Step	Infant (under 1 year)	Child (1–8 years)	Adult (over 8 years)
1. Check for responsiveness.	Stimulate to check response.	"Are you okay"—Tap shoulder	
2. If unresponsive, call 9-1-1.	Send someone to call. Give 5 cycles of CPR before calling yourself if alone.		Send someone to call. Call immediately if alone.
3. If unresponsive: Open airway.	Head tilt–chin lift (but do not overextend neck)	Head tilt–chin lift	
4. Check breathing.	Look, listen, feel for breathing.		
5. If not breathing: Give 2 breaths, watch chest rise.	Use barrier device or cover mouth, nose, or stoma. Each breath lasts 1 second.		
6. If chest does not rise with first breath: Reposition airway and try again.	Each breath lasts 1 second.		
7. Start chest compressions.	For compressions use two fingers just below line between nipples.	For compressions use one or two hands midway between nipples.	For compressions use both hands, one on top of other, midway between nipples.
Compression depth	Compress chest one-third to one-half of chest depth.		Compress chest 1½–2 inches.
Compression rate and ratio of compressions to breaths	Compress at rate of 100/minute—30 compressions per 2 breaths.		
8. Continue CPR until AED arrives, victim begins to move, or a professional rescuer takes over.	Continue cycles of 30 compressions and 2 breaths. Limit the time between the last compression and the first breath in each cycle to less than or equal to 10 seconds.		

(continued)

Step	Infant (under 1 year)	Child (1–8 years)	Adult (over 8 years)
9. Use AED when available (if victim is unresponsive and not breathing).	Not recommended.	Use pediatric electrode pads if available.	Use adult AED electrode pads
10. If victim begins to move and is breathing, put in recovery position.	Hold infant and monitor breathing.	Lay victim on side in recovery position and monitor breathing.	

3 Bleeding and Wound Care

Many injuries cause external or internal bleeding. Bleeding may be minor or life threatening. In addition to knowing how to control bleeding in a child, you should know how to care for different kinds of wounds and how to apply dressings and bandages.

TYPES OF EXTERNAL BLEEDING

There are three types of external bleeding (**Figure 3-1**):

- **Bleeding from injured arteries** is generally more serious and is more likely with deep injuries. The blood is bright red, and may spurt from the wound, and blood loss can be very rapid. This bleeding needs to be controlled immediately.
- **Bleeding from injured veins** is generally slower and steady but can still be serious. The blood is dark red and flows steadily rather than spurting. This bleeding is usually easier to control.
- **Bleeding from capillaries** occurs with shallow cuts or scrapes and often stops soon by itself. The wound still needs attention to prevent infection.

CONTROLLING EXTERNAL BLEEDING

For minor bleeding, clean and dress the wound (as described later). Usually the bleeding stops by itself or with light pressure on the dressing. For more serious bleeding, give first aid *immediately* to stop the bleeding.

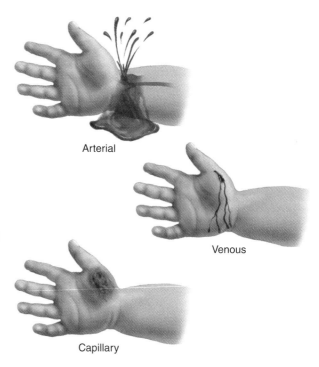

Arterial

Venous

Capillary

Figure 3-1 Types of external bleeding.

When You See

- Bleeding from a wound
- Blood on a child
- Signs of shock (see Chapter 4)

Do This First

1. Put on medical exam gloves or use another barrier to protect yourself from contact with the blood (such as dressings, a plastic bag, or the child's own hand).
2. Move aside any clothing and place a sterile dressing (or clean cloth) on the wound, then apply direct pressure on the wound with your hand.
3. If blood soaks through the dressing, do not remove the old dressing but put another dressing or cloth pad on top of it and keep applying pressure.
4. If possible, wrap a roller bandage around the limb to hold the dressings in place and apply pressure. Be careful not to cut off circulation to the limb with the many wraps of a roller bandage around the child's small limb.

Additional Care

- Call 9-1-1.
- Treat the child for shock if necessary (see Chapter 4).
- Do not remove the dressings/bandage. The wound will be cleaned later by medical personnel.
- Keep the child calm and distracted to ensure cooperation.

ALERT

Bleeding

Do not put pressure on an object in a wound.
Do not put pressure on the scalp if the skull may be injured.
Do not use a tourniquet to stop bleeding except as an extreme last resort (limb will likely be lost).

WOUND CARE

Wound care involves cleaning and dressing a wound to prevent infection and protect the wound so that healing can occur. Remember: *Do not waste time cleaning a wound that is severely bleeding. Controlling the bleeding is the priority.* Healthcare personnel will clean the wound as needed.

The main types of open wounds include the following:

- **Abrasions** occur when the top skin is scraped off. Foreign material may be present in the wound that can cause infection (**Figure 3-2**).
- **Lacerations**, or cuts, may be straight-edged (incision) or jagged, and may cause heavy bleeding (**Figure 3-3**).
- **Punctures** of the skin are caused by a sharp object penetrating down into the skin and possibly deeper tissues and are more likely to trap foreign material in the body (**Figure 3-4**).
- **Avulsions** are areas of skin or other tissue torn partially from the body, like a flap (**Figure 3-5**).

Other special wounds are described in the following pages.

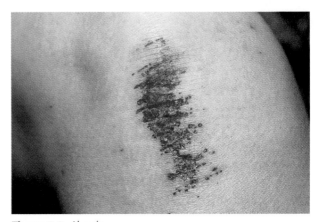

Figure 3-2 Abrasion.

Perform the Skill

Controlling Bleeding

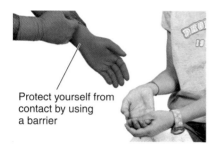

Protect yourself from contact by using a barrier

1 Put on gloves.

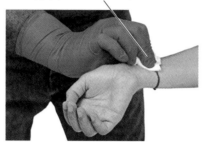

Apply pressure directly on wound

2 Place a sterile dressing on the wound and apply direct pressure with your hand.

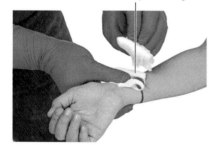

Do not remove a bloody dressing

3 If needed, put another dressing or cloth pad on top of the first and keep applying pressure.

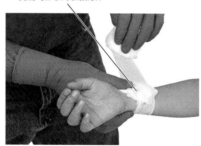

Make sure bandage is tight enough to apply pressure but not so tight it cuts off circulation

4 Apply a roller bandage to keep pressure on the wound.

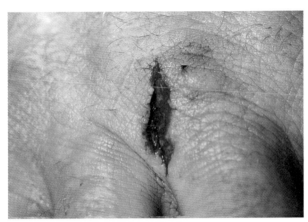

Figure 3-3 Laceration.

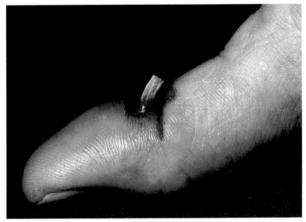

Figure 3-4 Puncture.

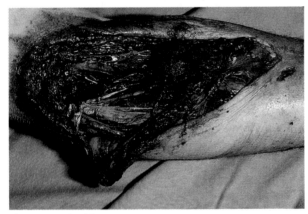

Figure 3-5 Avulsion.

When You See

- An open wound

Do This First

1. Gently wash the wound with soap and water to remove dirt. Let clean tap water run in and over the wound for at least 5 minutes to flush it clean.
2. Use a gauze pad or tweezers to remove any large particles.
3. Pat the area dry. With abrasions only, apply an antibiotic ointment (follow your childcare center's policy).
4. Cover the wound with a sterile dressing and bandage (or adhesive bandage with nonstick pad).

Additional Care

- If stitches may be needed (see later section), or if the child does not have a current tetanus vaccination, seek medical attention.
- Change the dressing daily or if it becomes wet. (If a dressing sticks to the wound, soak it in water first.) Advise the child's parents or caretakers to seek medical attention if the wound later looks infected.
- Keep the child calm and distracted to ensure cooperation.

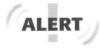

ALERT

Wound Cleaning

Do not try to clean a major wound after controlling bleeding—it may start bleeding again. Healthcare personnel will clean the wound as needed.
Do not use alcohol, hydrogen peroxide, or iodine on the wound.
Avoid breathing on the wound.

Cleaning Wounds

Unless the wound is very large or bleeding seriously, or the child has other injuries needing attention, clean the wound to help prevent infection. Wash your hands first and wear gloves if available.

Wound Infection

Any wound can become infected. The child then needs medical attention. The signs and symptoms of a wound infection include the following (**Figure 3-6**):

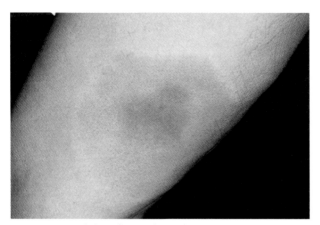

Figure 3-6 An infected wound.

- Wound area is red, swollen, and warm
- Pain
- Pus
- Fever
- Red streaks or trails on the skin near the wound are a sign the infection is spreading— see a healthcare provider immediately

Seek medical attention for any deep or puncture wound. With any deep or puncture wound, the risk of tetanus—a very serious infection—must be considered. Children are recommended to receive a series of tetanus vaccinations when young, followed by a booster in early adolescence and at least every 10 years thereafter. Some childcare centers and schools require children's vaccinations to be current, and your center may have a copy of this record. Parents or guardians should be advised when a tetanus shot may be needed.

Dressing Wounds

Dressings are put on wounds to help stop bleeding, prevent infection, and protect the wound while healing. First aid kits should include sealed sterile gauze dressings in many sizes. Adhesive strips such as Band-Aids are dressings combined with a bandage. If a sterile dressing is not available, use a clean, nonfluffy cloth as a dressing (**Figure 3-7**).

After washing and drying the wound, apply the dressing this way:

1. Wash your hands and wear gloves.
2. Choose a dressing larger than the wound.

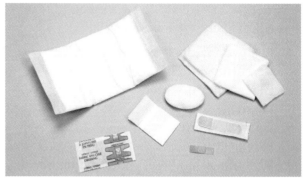

Figure 3-7 Variety of dressings.

3. Carefully lay the dressing on the wound (do not slide it on from the side).
4. If blood seeps through, do not remove the dressing but add more dressings on top.
5. Apply a bandage to hold the dressing in place (see later section on bandaging).

When to Seek Medical Attention

Remember to call 9-1-1 for severe bleeding. In addition, a child should see a healthcare provider as soon as possible in these situations:

- Bleeding is not easily controlled
- Any deep or large wound
- Significant wounds on the face
- Signs and symptoms that the wound is infected
- Any bite from an animal or human
- Foreign object or material embedded in the wound
- Any uncertainty about the child's tetanus vaccination
- The child may need stitches within hours for:
  - Cuts on the face or hands when the edges do not close together
  - Gaping wounds
  - Cuts longer than 1 inch

Special Wounds

Puncture Wounds

Puncture wounds have a greater risk of infection because often they bleed less and therefore germs may not be flushed out. In addition to routine wound care, take the following steps:

1. Remove any small objects or dirt but not larger impaled objects (see next section).
2. Gently press on wound edges to promote bleeding.
3. Do not put any medication inside or over the puncture wound.
4. Wash the wound well with running water directed at the puncture site.
5. Dress the wound and seek medical attention.

Impaled Objects

Removing an object from a wound could cause more injury and bleeding. Leave it in place and dress the wound around it.

1. Control bleeding by applying direct pressure at the sides of the object.
2. Dress the wound around the object.
3. Pad the object in place with large dressings or folded cloths.
4. Support the object while bandaging it in place.
5. Seek medical attention.

Amputation

In an amputation injury a body part has been severed from the body. Control the bleeding and care for the wound first. Call 9-1-1 and give care for shock as needed. Then recover and care for the amputated part. Use the following steps:

1. Wrap the severed part in dry sterile gauze. Do not wash it.
2. Place the part in a plastic bag and seal it.
3. Place the sealed bag in another bag or container with ice. Do not let the part touch ice directly, and do not surround it with ice (**Figure 3-8**).
4. Make sure the severed part is given to the responding crew or taken with the child to the emergency room.

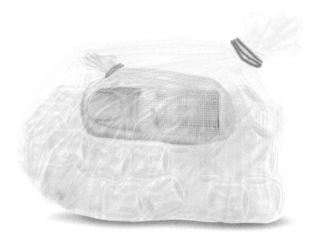

Figure 3-8 Keep amputated part cold but not directly touching ice.

Genital Injuries

Provide privacy for a child with bleeding or injury in the genital area. Follow these guidelines:

- Use direct pressure to control external bleeding.
- For injured testicles, provide support with a towel between the legs like a diaper.
- Call 9-1-1 for severe or continuing bleeding or significant pain or swelling. See Chapter 12 for steps to take if you suspect the possibility of sexual abuse.

Head and Face Wounds

Injuries to a child's head or face may require special first aid. The following sections list guidelines for these special injuries.

With any significant injury to the head, the child may also have a neck or spinal injury (see Chapter 6). If you suspect a spinal injury, be careful not to move the child's head while giving first aid for head and face wounds.

Skull Injuries

If the child is bleeding from the scalp, consider the additional possibility of a skull fracture if the child had a blow to the head.

When You See

- A deformed area of the skull
- A depressed area in the bone felt during the physical examination
- Blood or fluid from the ears or nose
- Object impaled in the skull

Do This First

1. If the child is unresponsive, check for breathing.
2. Do not clean the wound, press on it, or remove an impaled object.
3. Cover the wound with a sterile dressing.
4. If there is significant bleeding, apply pressure only around the edges of the wound, not on the wound itself.
5. Do not move the child unnecessarily, since there may also be a spinal injury.

Additional Care

- Call 9-1-1 and stay with the child.
- Because of the risk of a spinal injury, do not put the child in the recovery position.
- Seek medical attention if the child later experiences nausea and vomiting, persistent headache, drowsiness or disorientation, stumbling or lack of coordination, or problems with speech or vision.
- Keep the child calm and distracted to ensure cooperation.

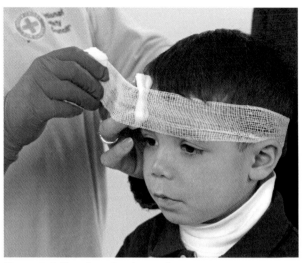

Figure 3-9 Dressing a head wound.

Do This First

1. Replace any skin flaps and cover the wound with a sterile dressing.
2. Use direct pressure to control bleeding.
3. Put a roller or triangle bandage around the child's head to secure the dressing (**Figure 3-9**).

Additional Care

- Position the child with head and shoulders raised to help control bleeding.
- If the wound was caused by a blow to the head or the wound may require stitches, the child should see a healthcare provider.
- Keep the child calm and distracted to ensure cooperation.

Head Wounds Without Suspected Skull Fracture

When You See

- Bleeding from the head
- No sign of skull fracture

Eye Injuries

Eye injuries can be serious because vision may be affected.

For a blow to the eye:

1. If the eye is bleeding or leaking fluid, call 9-1-1 immediately. Cover the injured eye with a paper cup bandaged or taped in place.

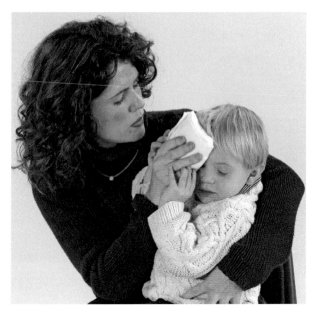

Figure 3-10 Blow to eye.

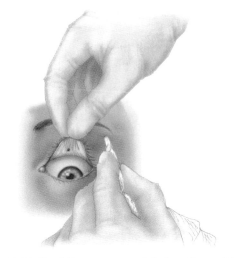

Figure 3-11 Carefully remove a particle from the eyelid.

2. If the eye is not bleeding or leaking fluid, put a cold pack over the eye for 15 minutes to ease pain and reduce swelling, but do not put pressure on the eye (**Figure 3-10**). If the child is wearing a contact lens, do not remove it.
3. Have the child lie still and also cover the uninjured eye. Movement of the uninjured eye causes movement of the injured one.
4. Seek medical attention if pain persists or vision is affected in any way.

For a large object embedded in the eye:

1. Do not remove the object. Stabilize it in place with dressings or bulky cloth.
2. Cover both eyes because movement of the uninjured one causes movement of the injured one.
3. Call 9-1-1 immediately.

For dirt or a small particle in the eye:

1. Do not let the child rub the eye.
2. Gently pull the upper eyelid out and down over the lower eyelid.
3. If the particle remains, gently flush the eye with water from a medicine dropper or water glass. Have the child hold his or her

head with the affected eye lower than the other so that water does not flow into the unaffected eye.
4. If the particle remains and is visible, carefully try to remove it with a sterile dressing. Lift the upper eyelid and swab its underside if you see the particle (**Figure 3-11**).
5. If the particle still remains or the child has any vision problems or pain, cover the eye with a sterile dressing and seek medical attention. Also cover the uninjured eye, because movement of the uninjured eye causes movement of the injured one.

For a chemical or substance splashed in the eye:

1. Rinse the eye with running water for 20 minutes. Have the child hold his or her head with the affected eye lower than the other so that water does not flow into the unaffected eye (see Chapter 5).
2. Call the Poison Control Center to determine what medical care may be needed.

Ear Injuries

With bleeding from the external ear, control the bleeding with direct pressure and dress the wound. For bleeding from within the ear, follow these guidelines:

When You See

- Bleeding inside the ear
- Signs of pain
- Possible deafness

Do This First

1. If the blood looks watery (which could mean a skull fracture) or the bleeding results from a blow to the head, call 9-1-1.
2. Help the child to sit up, tilting the affected ear lower to let blood drain out.
3. Cover the ear with a loose sterile dressing, but do not apply pressure.
4. Seek medical attention immediately.

Additional Care

- Keep the ear covered to reduce the risk of infection.
- Keep the child calm and distracted to ensure cooperation.

ALERT

Ear Wound

Do not plug the ear closed to try to stop bleeding.

Nosebleed

A nosebleed can be alarming because it often occurs suddenly and may seem to bleed heavily.

When You See

- Blood coming from either or both nostrils
- Blood possibly running from back of nose down into the mouth or throat

Do This First

1. Have the child sit and tilt his or her head slightly forward with the mouth open. Carefully remove any object you see in the nose.

2. Wearing gloves, pinch the child's nostrils together just below the bridge of the nose and hold for 10 minutes; an older child may be able to hold his or her nostrils pinched closed. Ask the child to breathe through the mouth and not speak, swallow, cough, or sniff.
3. If the child is gasping or choking on blood in the throat, call 9-1-1.
4. After 10 minutes, release the pressure slowly. Pinch the nostrils again for another 10 minutes if bleeding continues.
5. Place a cold compress on the bridge of the nose (**Figure 3-12**).

Additional Care

- Seek medical attention if:
  - bleeding continues after two attempts to control bleeding,
  - you suspect the nose is broken, or
  - the child is known to have high blood pressure.
- Have the child rest for a few hours and avoid rubbing, picking at, or blowing the nose.
- Keep the child calm and distracted to ensure cooperation.

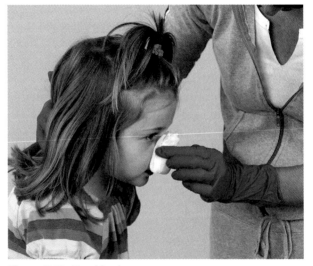

Figure 3-12 Nosebleed care.

Nosebleed
Do not tilt the child's head backward.
Do not have the child lie down.

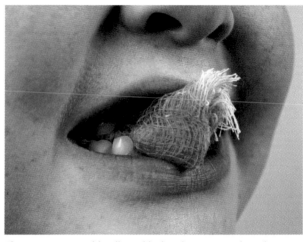

Figure 3-13 Stop bleeding with dressing over tooth socket.

Broken Nose

When You See

- Obvious deformity of the nose
- Swelling
- Blood coming from either or both nostrils

Do This First

1. Have the child sit and tilt his or her head slightly forward with the mouth open.
2. If bleeding is significant, try to stop the bleeding by pinching the nostrils closed as for a nosebleed.
3. Call 9-1-1 or seek medical attention.

Mouth and Tooth Injuries

For a tooth knocked out:

1. Have the child sit with head tilted forward to let blood drain out.
2. To control bleeding, fold or roll gauze into a pad and place it over the tooth socket. Have the child bite down to put pressure on the pad (**Figure 3-13**).
3. Save the tooth, which may be reimplanted if the child sees a dentist within the first hour after the injury. Touching only the tooth's crown, rinse it if dirty. Put the tooth in a container of milk, or use a commercial tooth saver kit.

4. Get the child and the tooth to a dentist immediately. (Most dentists have 24-hour emergency call numbers.)

For other bleeding in the mouth:

1. Have the child sit with head tilted forward to let blood drain out.
2. **For a wound penetrating the lip:** Put a rolled dressing between the lip and the gum. Hold a second dressing against the outside lip.
3. **For a bleeding tongue:** Put a dressing on the wound and apply pressure.
4. Do not rinse the mouth (this may prevent clotting).
5. Do not let the child swallow blood, which may cause vomiting.
6. Do not let the child drink anything warm for several hours.
7. Seek medical attention if bleeding is severe or does not stop.

BANDAGES

Bandages are used for covering a dressing, keeping the dressing on a wound, and applying pressure to stop bleeding. Because only dressings touch the wound itself, bandages need to be clean but not necessarily sterile. As described in Chapter 7, bandages are also used to support or immobilize an injury to bones, joints, or muscles and to reduce swelling.

Types of Bandages

Your first aid kit should contain a variety of bandages. All the following are examples of bandages (**Figure 3-14**):

- Adhesive compresses or strips for small wounds that combine a dressing with an adhesive bandage
- Adhesive tape rolls (cloth, plastic, paper)
- Tubular bandages for finger or toe
- Elastic bandages
- Cloth roller bandages
- Triangular bandages (or folded square cloths)
- Any cloth or other material improvised to meet purposes of bandaging

Guidelines for Bandaging

1. To put pressure on a wound to stop bleeding or to prevent swelling of an

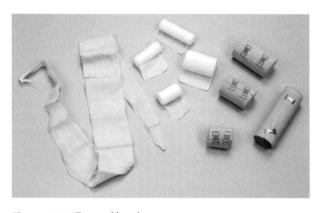

Figure 3-14 Types of bandages.

injury, apply the bandage firmly—but not so tightly that it cuts off circulation. With a bandage around a limb, check the fingers or toes for color, warmth, and sensation (normal touch, not tingling) to make sure circulation is not cut off. If there are signs of reduced circulation, unwrap the bandage and reapply it less tightly.

2. Since swelling continues after many injuries, keep checking the tightness of the bandage. Swelling may make a loose bandage tight enough to cut off circulation.

3. With a bandaged wound, be sure the bandage is secure enough that the dressing will not move and expose the wound to possible contamination.

4. With elastic and roller bandages, anchor the first end and tie, tape, or pin the ending section in place.

5. Use a nonelastic roller bandage to make a pressure bandage around a limb to control bleeding and protect the wound.

6. An elastic roller bandage is used to support a joint and prevent swelling. At the wrist or ankle a figure-eight wrap is used.

INTERNAL BLEEDING

Internal bleeding is any bleeding within the body in which the blood does not escape from an open wound. A closed wound may have minor local bleeding in the skin and other superficial tissue, causing a bruise. A more serious injury of the torso can cause deeper organs to bleed severely. This bleeding, although unseen, can be life threatening. (See also Chapter 6 on closed abdominal wounds.)

Perform the Skill

Applying a Pressure Bandage

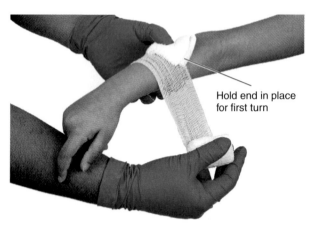

Hold end in place for first turn

1 Anchor the starting end of the bandage below the wound dressing.

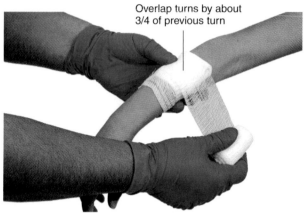

Overlap turns by about 3/4 of previous turn

2 Make several circular turns, then overlap turns.

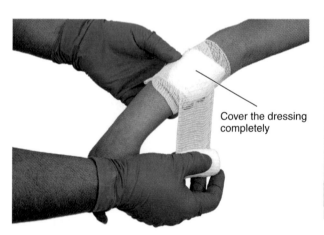

Cover the dressing completely

3 Work up the limb.

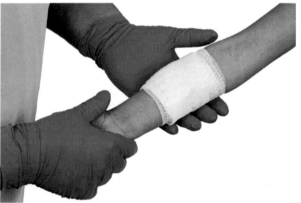

4 Tape or tie the end of the bandage in place.

Perform the Skill

Applying a Roller Bandage

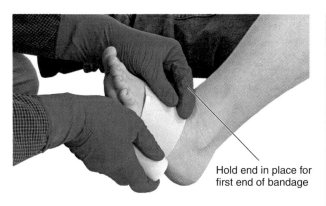

Hold end in place for
first end of bandage

1 Anchor the starting end of the bandage.

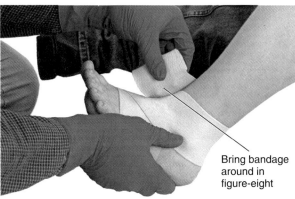

Bring bandage
around in
figure-eight

2 Turn bandage diagonally across top of foot and
around ankle.

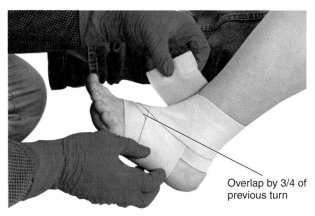

Overlap by 3/4 of
previous turn

3 Continue with overlapping figure-eight turns.

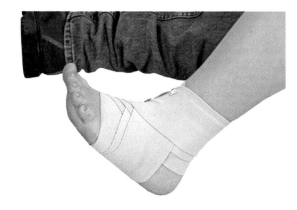

4 Fasten end of bandage with clips, tape, or safety
pins.

For simple closed wounds:

When You See

- Bruising
- Signs of pain

Do This First

1. Check for signs and symptoms of a fracture or sprain (see Chapter 7) and give appropriate first aid.
2. Put ice or a cold pack on the area to control bleeding, reduce swelling, and reduce pain.
3. With an arm or leg, wrap the area with an elastic bandage. Keep the part raised to help reduce swelling.

Additional Care

- Seek medical attention if you suspect a more serious injury such as a fracture or sprain.
- Keep the child calm and distracted to ensure cooperation.

For internal bleeding:

When You See

- Abdomen is tender, swollen, bruised, or hard
- Blood vomited or coughed up, or present in urine
- Cool, clammy skin, may be pale or bluish
- Thirst
- Possible confusion, light-headedness

Do This First

1. Lay the child down on the back with legs raised 8 to 12 inches.
2. Call 9-1-1.
3. Be alert for vomiting. Put a child who vomits or becomes unresponsive in the recovery position.
4. Maintain the child's body temperature.

Additional Care

- Calm and reassure the child.
- If the child becomes unresponsive, monitor breathing and give basic life support (BLS) as needed.
- Treat for shock (see Chapter 4).

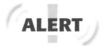

ALERT

Internal Bleeding

Do not give the child anything to drink even if he or she is very thirsty.

Chapter

4 Shock

Shock is a dangerous condition in which not enough oxygen-rich blood is reaching vital organs in the body. The brain, heart, and other organs need a continual supply of oxygen. Anything that happens to or in the body that significantly reduces blood flow can cause shock.

Shock is a life-threatening emergency. It may develop quickly or gradually. Always call 9-1-1 for a child in shock.

CAUSES OF SHOCK

- *Severe bleeding* causes shock when there is not enough blood circulating in the body to bring required oxygen to vital organs. This is the most common cause of shock in children. With internal injuries, it may not be obvious a child is bleeding inside.
- *Heart problems,* like a heart attack or heart rhythm problem, cause shock when the heart cannot pump enough blood to meet the body's needs.
- *Nervous system injuries,* such as those caused by neck or spine injuries, can affect the heart or blood vessels in ways that prevent adequate blood from reaching vital organs.

Many other types of injuries can also cause some degree of shock. Some specific examples are as follows:

- Dehydration (such as may occur in heatstroke or with severe vomiting or diarrhea)
- Serious infections
- Severe burns
- Allergic reactions (see later section on Anaphylaxis)
- Heart failure

FIRST AID FOR SHOCK

Shock has various signs and symptoms depending on its cause and severity. A child with any serious injury should be assumed to be at risk of shock, even if you do not see all these signs and symptoms (**Figure 4-1**).

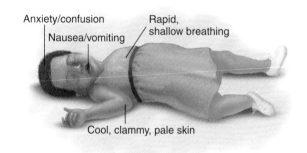

Anxiety/confusion
Nausea/vomiting
Rapid, shallow breathing
Cool, clammy, pale skin

Figure 4-1 Signs of shock.

When You See

- Anxiety, confusion, agitation, or restlessness
- Dizziness, light-headedness
- Cool, clammy or sweating, pale or bluish skin
- Rapid, shallow breathing
- Thirst
- Nausea, vomiting
- Changing levels of responsiveness

Do This First

1. Give basic life support (BLS) and care for life-threatening injuries.
2. Call 9-1-1.
3. Have the child lie on his or her back and raise the legs about 8 to 12 inches (unless the child may have a spine injury). Loosen any tight clothing (**Figure 4-2**).
4. Try to maintain the child's normal body temperature. If lying on the ground, put a coat or blanket under the child. If in doubt, keep the child warm with a blanket or coat over his or her body (**Figure 4-3**).

Additional Care

- Stay with the child and offer reassurance and comfort.
- Put an unresponsive child (if spinal injury is not suspected) in the recovery position.
- Keep bystanders from crowding around the child.

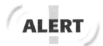

ALERT

Shock

Do not let a child in shock eat or drink. Note that sweating in a child in shock is not necessarily a sign of being too warm. If in doubt, it is better to ensure the child's body temperature by keeping the child warm.

ANAPHYLAXIS

Anaphylaxis is a severe allergic reaction, also called anaphylactic shock. It is a life-threatening emergency because the child's airway may swell, making breathing difficult or impossible. Always call 9-1-1 for an anaphylaxis emergency. Common causes of anaphylaxis include:

- Certain drugs (such as penicillins, sulfa)
- Certain foods (such as peanuts, shellfish, eggs)
- Insect stings and bites (such as bees or wasps)

Some older children who know they have a severe allergy may carry an emergency epinephrine kit such as an EpiPen-Jr. This medication can temporarily stop the anaphylactic reaction. Ask the child about this and help him or her open the kit. Follow your childcare center's policy to use the kit as needed. The EpiPen-Jr is removed from its case and the cap removed. The tip is then jabbed into the muscle of the outer part of the thigh and held there 5 to 10 seconds (**Figure 4-4**). The injection site is then massaged for a few seconds. The

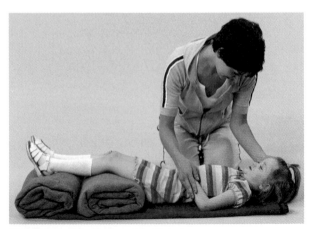

Figure 4-2 Raise the legs 8 to 12 inches.

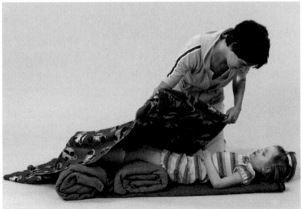

Figure 4-3 Try to maintain the child's normal body temperature.

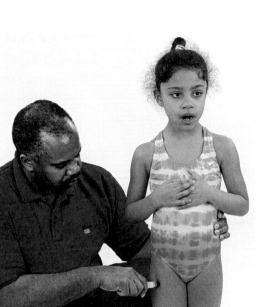

Figure 4-4 Using an EpiPen-Jr.

effects of the emergency epinephrine may last 10 to 20 minutes. A second dose may be needed and can be given 10 minutes after the first dose.

When You See

- Difficulty breathing, wheezing
- Complaints of tightness in throat or chest
- Swelling of the face and neck, puffy eyes
- Red, blotchy skin
- Anxiety, agitation
- Nausea, vomiting
- Changing levels of responsiveness

Do This First

1. Call 9-1-1.
2. Give BLS as needed.
3. Help the child use his or her epinephrine kit if available.
4. Help the child sit up in position of easiest breathing (Figure 4-5).

Additional Care

- Stay with the child and offer reassurance and comfort.
- Put a breathing unresponsive child (if spinal injury is not suspected) in the recovery position.

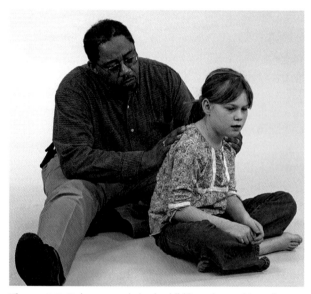

Figure 4-5 Help an anaphylactic child into the position of easiest breathing.

Chapter

5 Burns

Burns of the skin or deeper tissues may be caused by heat, chemicals, or electricity. Mild heat burns and sunburn may need only simple first aid, but severe burns are a medical emergency. Burns are more common in children because many children have not learned safety guidelines around fire or heat sources.

HEAT BURNS

Heat burns may be caused by flames, contact with steam or any hot object, or sun exposure. The severity of a burn depends on the amount of damage to the skin and other tissues under the skin.

Put Out the Fire!

If a child's clothing is on fire, have him or her **stop, drop, and roll** (**Figure 5-1**). Use water to put out any flames. Even when the fire is out, the skin will keep burning if it is still hot, so cool the burn area with water immediately, except with very severe burns. Also remove the child's clothing and any jewelry, if possible without further injuring the child, because these items may still be hot and continue to burn the child.

How Bad Is the Burn?

- **First-degree burns** (also called superficial burns) damage only the skin's outer layer, like a sunburn. These are typically minor burns and usually heal by themselves.
- **Second-degree burns** (also called partial-thickness burns) damage the skin's deeper layers. When small they may not be too serious, but larger second-degree burns require medical attention.
- **Third-degree burns** (also called full-thickness burns) damage the skin all the way through and may burn the muscle or other tissues. These are medical emergencies (**Figure 5-2**).

Also important is the location of the burn on the body. Burns on the face, genitals, or hands or feet generally are more serious and require medical care.

First-Degree Burns (Including Sunburn)

When You See

- Skin is red, dry, and painful (**Figure 5-3**)
- May be some swelling
- Skin not broken

Do This First

1. Stop the burning by removing the heat source.
2. Cool the burned area with cold water. Immerse a small area in a sink or bucket, or cover a

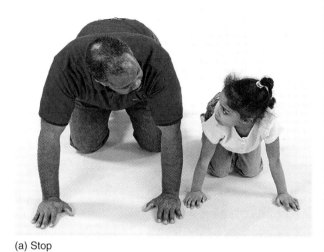

(a) Stop

larger area (but not most of the body) with wet cloths until pain is relieved.

3. Remove clothing and jewelry or any other constricting item before the area swells.

4. Protect the burn from friction or pressure.

Additional Care

- Aloe vera gel can be used on the skin for comfort (follow your childcare center's policy).
- Give the child cool water to drink.
- Follow your childcare center's policy on giving acetaminophen or ibuprofen for pain (parental permission required).

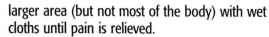

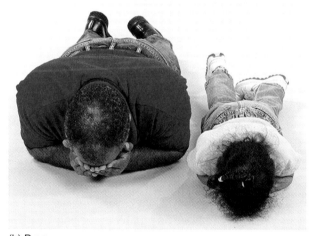

(b) Drop

ALERT

Burn

Do not put butter on a burn. Do not use ice on a burn because even though it may relieve pain, the cold can actually cause additional damage to the skin.

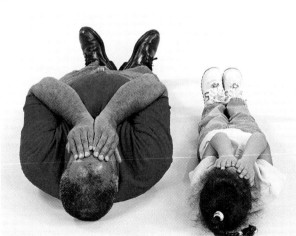

(c) Roll

Figure 5-1 Teach children to stop, drop, and roll.

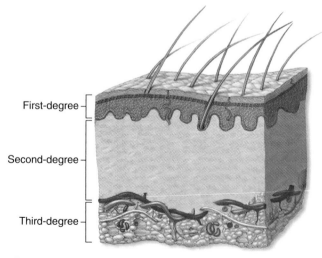

Figure 5-2 Depth of a burn.

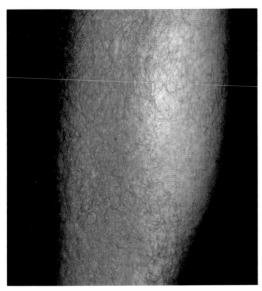

Figure 5-3 First-degree burn.

Second-Degree Burns

When You See

- Skin is swollen and red, may be blotchy or streaked
- Blisters that may be weeping clear fluid (**Figure 5-4**)
- Signs of significant pain

Do This First

1. Stop the burning by removing the heat source.

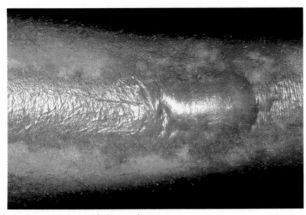

Figure 5-4 Second-degree burn.

2. Cool the burned area with cold water. Immerse a small area in a sink or bucket, or cover a larger area (but not most of the body) with wet cloths for at least 10 minutes or until the area is free of pain even after removal from the water.
3. Remove clothing and jewelry from the area before the area swells.
4. Put a dressing over the burn to protect the area, but keep it loose and do not tape it to the skin.

Additional Care

- For large burns or burns on the face, genitals, hands, or feet, seek medical attention. A young child with a second-degree burn more than an inch across needs medical attention.
- Follow your childcare center's policy to contact the child's parents.

ALERT

Second-Degree Burn

Do not break skin blisters! This could cause an infection. Be gentle when covering the area. Do not remove any material sticking to the burned area.

Third-Degree Burns

When You See

- Skin damage, charred skin, or white leathery skin (**Figure 5-5**)
- May have signs and symptoms of shock (pale, clammy skin; nausea and vomiting; fast breathing)

Do This First

1. Stop the burning by removing the heat source.
2. Cool surrounding first- and second-degree burns only.

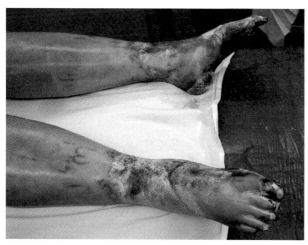

Figure 5-5 Third-degree burn.

3. Remove clothing and jewelry before the area swells.
4. Call 9-1-1.
5. Prevent shock: have the child lie down, elevate the legs, and maintain normal body temperature.
6. Carefully cover the burn with a dressing. Do not apply a cream or ointment.

Additional Care

- Watch the child's breathing and be ready to give basic life support (BLS) if needed.
- Do not give the child anything to drink.

ALERT

Third-Degree Burn

With third-degree burns do not cool more than 10% of the child's body with water because of the risk of hypothermia and shock. Do not touch the burn or put anything on it. Do not remove any material sticking to the burned area.

Smoke Inhalation

Inhaling very hot air or smoke can burn the airway from the mouth to the lungs. This can be a medical emergency. Because the signs and symptoms from smoke inhalation may not become obvious for up to 48 hours after exposure, any child thought to have inhaled smoke should see a healthcare provider.

When You See

- Smoke visible in area
- Coughing, wheezing, hoarse voice
- Possible burned area on face or chest
- Difficulty breathing

Do This First

1. Get the child to fresh air, or fresh air to the child.
2. Call 9-1-1.
3. Help the child into a position for easy breathing.

Additional Care

- Put an unresponsive child in the recovery position.
- Loosen any clothing around the neck.
- Be ready to give BLS if needed.

CHEMICAL BURNS

Many strong chemicals found in the home, childcare centers, and other settings can "burn" the skin on contact (**Figure 5-6**). See Chapters 15 and 16 for steps you can take to prevent children from contacting substances that can cause chemical burns. See Chapter 9 for chemicals on or in the mouth.

Sometimes the burn develops slowly, and in some cases the child may not even be aware

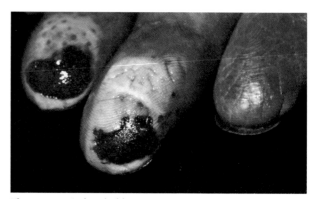

Figure 5-6 A chemical burn.

of the burn at first. Both acids and alkalis, and liquids and solids can cause serious burns. Since the chemical reaction can continue as long as the substance is on the skin, you must flush it off with water as soon as possible.

When You See

- A chemical on the child's skin or clothing
- Complaints of pain or a burning sensation
- Skin redness or discoloration, blistering or peeling
- A spilled substance on or around an unresponsive child
- A smell of fumes in the air

Do This First

1. With a dry chemical, first brush it off the child's skin. (Wear medical exam gloves to prevent contact with the substance yourself.)
2. With a spilled liquid giving off fumes, move the child or ventilate the area.
3. Wash off the area as quickly as possible with running water for at least 30 minutes. Use a sink, hose, or even a shower to flush the whole area of contact.
4. Remove clothing and jewelry from the burn area.
5. Call 9-1-1 for large or deep chemical burns, or any burns on the child's face or head, hands or feet, or genital area.

Additional Care

- If chemicals were spilled in a confined area, leave the area with the child because of the risk of fumes.
- Put a dry dressing over the burn.
- A child with any chemical burn needs medical attention.

Chemicals in Eye

If a chemical splashes into a child's eye, flush the eye immediately with running water and continue for 20 minutes. If the child is wearing contact lenses, have him or her remove them.

Tilt the child's head so that the water runs away from the face and not into the other eye. Call 9-1-1. After flushing, have the child hold a dressing over the eye until a healthcare provider is seen.

ELECTRICAL BURNS AND SHOCKS

Electrical burns may include:

- External burns caused by the heat of electricity
- Electrical injuries caused by electricity flowing through the body

External burns resulting from heat or flames caused by electricity are cared for the same as heat burns. Electrical injuries may cause only minor external burns where the electricity both entered and left the body (called entrance and exit wounds). But electricity flowing through the body can stop the heart and cause other serious injuries.

When You See

- A source of electricity near the child: bare wires, power cords, an electrical device
- Burned area of skin, possibly both entrance and exit wounds (Figure 5-7)
- Changing responsiveness

Do This First

1. Do not touch the child until you know the area is safe. Unplug or turn off the power.
2. With an unresponsive child, check for breathing and give BLS as needed.
3. Call 9-1-1.
4. Care for the burn (stop the burning, cool the area, remove clothing and jewelry, cover the burn).
5. Prevent shock by having the child lie down, elevate the legs, and maintain normal body temperature.

Additional Care

- Keep an unresponsive child in the recovery position and monitor breathing until help arrives.

ALERT

Electrical Shock

Do not touch a child you think has had an electrical shock until you are certain the power is turned off or the child is well away from the power source. Turn off the circuit breaker and call 9-1-1. Note that electrical burns can cause massive internal injuries even when the external burn may look minor.

LIGHTNING STRIKES

Lightning strikes often cause serious injury. In addition to burns, the electrical shock may affect the heart and brain and cause temporary blindness or deafness, unresponsiveness or seizures, bleeding, bone fractures, and cardiac arrest. Call 9-1-1 immediately and give BLS, treating the most serious injuries first.

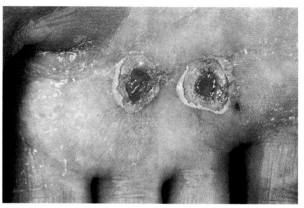

Figure 5-7　An electrical burn.

6 Serious Injuries

Many factors affect how serious a child's injury may be. As you have learned, injuries that threaten the child's airway, breathing, or circulation are life threatening. Severe bleeding is also very serious. This chapter describes some additional injuries in specific areas of the body that can be very serious for children and may become life threatening.

HEAD AND SPINAL INJURIES

Head injuries are common in children. Usually they are minor, such as a bump on the head (see Chapter 11), but with a more severe impact they may be serious. Any injury to a child's head may also injure the spine. Whenever you encounter a serious head injury, suspect a neck or spine injury also.

Skull Fractures

A skull fracture is life threatening. Call 9-1-1 immediately. Chapter 3 describes the signs and symptoms of a skull fracture and the first aid to give while waiting for help.

Brain Injuries

Brain injuries include bleeding, swelling, and concussion. A **concussion** is a temporary impairment of brain function and usually does not involve permanent damage. However, it is generally difficult to determine whether a child's injury is moderately or very serious, and the child may have a variety of signs and symptoms. Do not worry about trying to figure out what specifically is wrong with a head injury—just call 9-1-1 and give supportive care while waiting for help.

When You See

- Head wound suggesting there was a blow to the head
- Changing levels of responsiveness, drowsiness
- Difficulty being awakened
- Confusion, disorientation, memory loss about the injury
- Headache
- Dizziness
- Lack of coordination, clumsiness, abnormal speech
- Nausea, vomiting
- Unequal pupils (Figure 6-1)
- Convulsions

Do This First

For a responsive child:

1. Have the child lie down.
2. Keep the child still and help maintain the child's normal body temperature.
3. Call 9-1-1 and monitor the child's condition until help arrives.

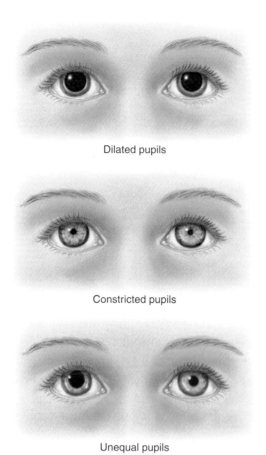

Dilated pupils

Constricted pupils

Unequal pupils

Figure 6-1 Check to see if a child's pupils are dilated, constricted, or unequal.

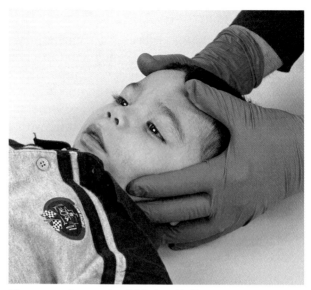

Figure 6-2 Support the child's head in line with his or her body for suspected spinal injury.

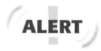

Brain Injury
Do not let the child eat or drink anything.
Do not give a pain medication.

For an unresponsive child:

1. Check the child's breathing without moving the child unless necessary. Assume there may be a spinal injury.
2. Control serious bleeding and cover any wounds with a dressing.
3. Call 9-1-1.
4. If the child vomits, move him or her into the recovery position. If you suspect a spinal injury, support the child's head and neck at all times.

Additional Care

- Support the neck, even in a responsive child, if you suspect a spinal injury (**Figure 6-2**).

Later Signs and Symptoms

In some cases after a blow to the head the child does not have the signs and symptoms listed earlier and does not receive medical care. Signs and symptoms appearing within 48 hours may indicate a more serious injury, however, including nausea and vomiting, severe or persistent headache, altered or changing responsiveness, problems with vision or speech, or seizures. The child needs medical attention immediately if any of these occurs following a head injury.

Infants

Because an infant's skull bones are not completely formed and not yet as strong as an older child's, any infant who experiences a blow to the head should be seen by a healthcare provider. Call 9-1-1 immediately if the infant has any of the signs and symptoms described earlier for a child, and monitor the infant's breathing.

Spinal Injuries

A fracture of the neck or back is a spinal injury. This injury may be life threatening and can cause permanent paralysis. It is very important not to move the child any more than necessary and to support the head and neck to prevent worsening of the injury. Do not let a child with a suspected spinal injury try to sit or stand up or move around, because any movement of the neck could damage nerves.

Suspect a spinal injury in these situations:

- A fall from a height (even a short height)
- A motor vehicle or bicycle crash
- A blow to the head or back
- A crushing injury of the head, neck, or back
- A diving injury

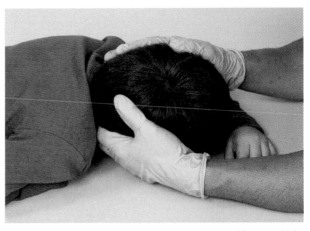

Figure 6-3 Support the head and neck in the position in which you find the child.

When You See

In a responsive child:
- Inability to move any body part
- Lack of sensation or tingling in hands or feet
- Deformed neck or back
- Breathing problems
- Headache

In an unresponsive child:
- Deformed neck or back
- Signs of blow to head or back
- Nature of the emergency suggests possible spinal injury

Do This First

1. Assess a responsive child:
   - Can the child move his or her fingers and toes?
   - Can the child feel you touch his or her hands and feet?
2. Stabilize the child's head and neck in the position in which you found the child (**Figure 6-3**).

3. Monitor the child's breathing and keep the airway open if necessary in an unresponsive child.
4. Have someone call 9-1-1.
5. For a long wait, or if you must leave the child to call 9-1-1, use padding or heavy objects on both sides of head to prevent movement.

Additional Care

- Reassure a responsive child and tell him or her not to move.
- Continue to monitor the child's breathing until help arrives.

Always support the child's head and neck in the position found. Move the child only if absolutely necessary, such as if a child lying on his or her back vomits. If this occurs, you must roll the child onto his or her side to let the mouth drain and allow breathing. The help of one or two others is necessary to keep the child's back and neck aligned during the move.

CHEST INJURIES

Serious chest injuries include broken ribs, objects impaled in the chest, and sucking chest wounds in which air passes in and out of the chest cavity.

Perform the Skill

Inline Stabilization

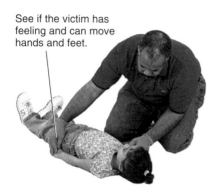

See if the victim has feeling and can move hands and feet.

1 Assess a responsive child for spinal injury.

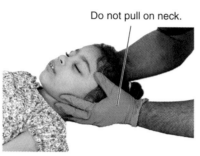

Do not pull on neck.

2 Hold the child's head with both hands to prevent movement of neck or spine. Have someone call 9-1-1.

3 Monitor the child's breathing.

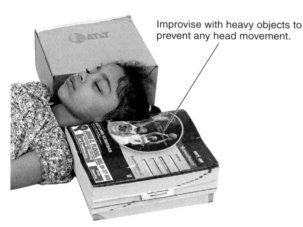

Improvise with heavy objects to prevent any head movement.

4 Use objects to maintain head support if needed.

These wounds can be life threatening if breathing is affected. Chest injuries may result from such things as:

- A motor vehicle crash
- A blow to the chest
- A fall from a height

The general signs and symptoms of a chest injury include:

- Breathing problems
- Severe pain
- Deformity of the chest
- Possibly coughing blood

Perform the Skill

Rolling a Child with Spinal Injury (Log Roll)

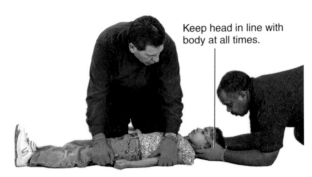

Keep head in line with body at all times.

1 Hold the child's head with your hands on both sides over ears.

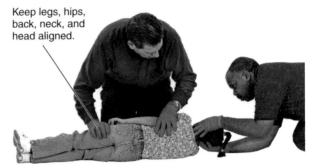

Keep legs, hips, back, neck, and head aligned.

2 The first aider at the child's head directs others to roll body as a unit.

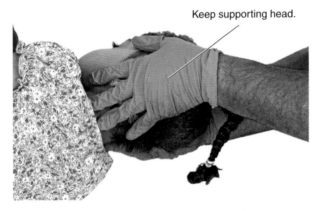

Keep supporting head.

3 Continue to support the child's head in the new position on his or her side.

Broken Ribs

When You See

- Signs of pain with deep breathing or movement
- Child holding ribs
- Shallow breathing

Do This First

1. Have child sit in position of easiest breathing.

2. Support the ribs with a pillow or soft padding (Figure 6-4). This can be loosely bandaged over the area and under the arm.

3. Call 9-1-1.

Additional Care

- Monitor the child's breathing while waiting for help, and provide BLS if needed.
- If needed, immobilize the arm with a sling and binder (see Chapter 7) to prevent movement and ease pain.

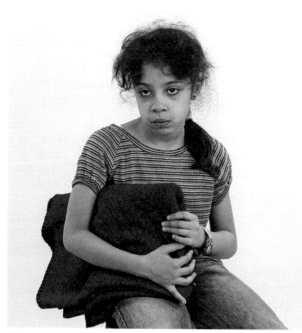

Figure 6-4 Support a rib fracture.

Impaled Object

Removing an impaled object from a child's chest could cause additional bleeding and breathing problems. If a child has an impaled object, leave it in place and seek medical attention.

When You See

- An object impaled in a chest wound

Do This First

1. Keep the child still. The child may be seated or lying down.
2. Use bulky dressings or cloth to stabilize the object.
3. Bandage the area around the object.
4. Call 9-1-1.

Additional Care

- Reassure the child.
- Monitor the child's breathing until help arrives.

ALERT

Chest Injury

Do not give the child anything to eat or drink.

Sucking Chest Wound

A sucking chest wound is an open wound in the chest caused by a penetrating injury. The wound lets air move in and out of the chest during breathing. This wound can be life threatening because breathing can be affected.

When You See

- Air moving in or out of a penetrating chest wound

Do This First

1. Put a thin sterile dressing over the wound.
2. Cover the dressing with a plastic bag or wrap to make an air-tight seal. As the child exhales, tape it in place on three sides, leaving one side untaped to let exhaled air escape.
3. Position the child lying down inclined toward the injured side.
4. Call 9-1-1.

Additional Care

- If the child's breathing becomes more difficult, remove the plastic seal to let air escape; then reapply it.
- Monitor the child's breathing until help arrives.

ABDOMINAL INJURIES

Abdominal injuries include closed and open wounds that result from a blow to the abdomen or a fall. These may involve internal and/or external bleeding, and organs may protrude from the wound. The child needs immediate medical care even if no significant injuries can be seen.

Closed Abdominal Injury

A closed abdominal injury can be life threatening because internal organs may have ruptured and there may be serious internal bleeding.

When You See

- Signs of severe pain, tenderness in area
- Bruising
- Swollen or rigid abdomen

Do This First

1. Carefully position the child on his or her back. Allow the child to bend the knees slightly if this eases the pain (support with a pillow under the knees).
2. Loosen any tight clothing.
3. Call 9-1-1.
4. Treat the child for shock.

Additional Care

- Continue to monitor the child's breathing until help arrives.

ALERT

Abdominal Injury

Do not let the child eat or drink.

Open Abdominal Wound

When You See

- Open abdominal wound
- Bleeding
- Organs possibly protruding from wound

Do This First

1. Lay the child on his or her back. Allow the child to bend the knees slightly if this eases the pain (support with a pillow under the knees).

2. Loosen any tight clothing.
3. If organs are protruding through the wound opening, do not try to push them back in. Cover the wound with a dressing moistened with sterile or clean water, or plastic wrap if water is unavailable.
4. Cover the moistened dressing with a large dry sterile dressing and tape it loosely in place.
5. Call 9-1-1.
6. Treat the child for shock.

Additional Care

- Continue to monitor the child's breathing until help arrives.

ALERT

Open Abdominal Wound

Do not push protruding organs back inside the abdomen, but keep them from drying out with a moist dressing or plastic covering.

PELVIC INJURIES

A broken pelvis may cause severe internal bleeding and organ damage. A broken pelvis can be a life-threatening injury.

When You See

- Signs of pain and tenderness around the hips
- Inability to walk or stand
- Signs and symptoms of shock

Do This First

1. Help the child lie on his or her back and bend knees slightly if this eases the pain (support with a pillow under the knees).
2. Immobilize the child's legs by placing padding between the thighs and ankles and then bandaging them together, unless this causes more pain (**Figure 6-5**).

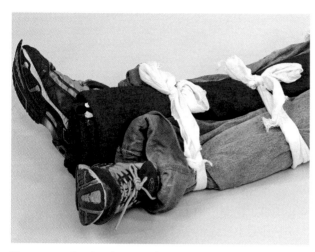

Figure 6-5 Bandage legs together for a pelvic injury.

3. Call 9-1-1.

4. Treat the child for shock.

Additional Care

- Continue to monitor the child's breathing until help arrives.

7 Bone, Joint, and Muscle Injuries

Injuries of the bones, joints, and muscles are among the most common injuries in children. Fractures are generally the most serious, although dislocations and sprains can also be very serious. Fortunately, most musculoskeletal injuries do not involve fractures or dislocations.

FRACTURES

A **fracture** is a broken bone. The bone may be completely broken with the pieces separated, or it may be only cracked. With a **closed fracture** the skin is not broken. With an **open fracture** there is an open wound at the fracture site, and bone may protrude through the wound (**Figure 7-1**). Bleeding can be severe with fractures of large bones, and organs nearby may also be injured.

When You See

- A deformed body part (compare to other side of body) (**Figure 7-2**)
- Signs of pain
- Swelling, discoloration of skin
- Inability to use the body part
- Bone exposed in a wound
- The child heard or felt a bone snap
- Possible signs and symptoms of shock

Do This First

1. Have the child rest and be still. Immobilize the area. With an extremity, also immobilize the joints above and below the fracture.
2. Call 9-1-1 for a large bone fracture. A child with a fractured hand or foot may be transported to the emergency department, following your childcare center's policy.
3. With an open fracture, cover the wound with a dressing and apply gentle pressure around the fracture area only if needed to control bleeding.

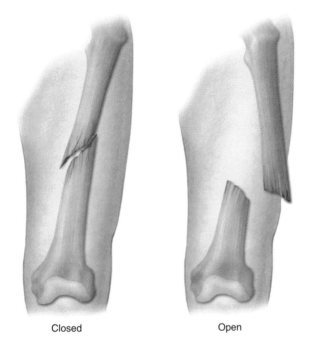

Closed   Open

Figure 7-1 Closed and open fractures.

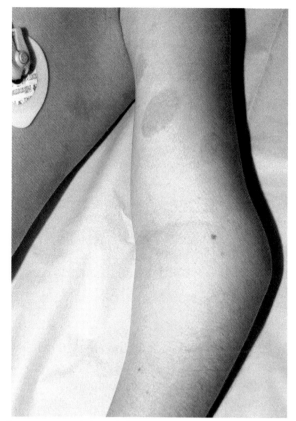

Figure 7-2 An obvious deformity may indicate a fracture.

4. Put ice or a cold pack on the area for 20 minutes, then at least 30 minutes off.

5. If help may be delayed or if the child is to be transported, use a splint to keep the area immobilized (see later section on splints). Elevate a splinted arm.

Additional Care

- Treat the child for shock as needed.
- Monitor the child's breathing.
- Remove clothing and jewelry if they may cut off circulation as swelling occurs.

ALERT

Fracture

Do not try to align the ends of a broken bone. Do not give the child anything to eat or drink.

Joint Injuries

Injuries to joints include dislocations and sprains. In a **dislocation,** one or more bones have been moved out of the normal position in a joint. A **sprain** is an injury to ligaments and other structures in a joint. Both kinds of joint injuries often look similar to a fracture.

Dislocations

It is not always possible to tell a dislocation from a closed fracture, but the first aid is very similar.

When You See

- The joint is deformed (compare to other side of body)
- Signs of pain
- Swelling
- Inability to use the body part

Do This First

1. Have the child rest. Immobilize the injured area in the position in which you find it.

2. Call 9-1-1. A child with a dislocated bone in the hand or foot may be transported to the emergency department, following your childcare center's policy.

3. Put ice or a cold pack on the area for 20 minutes, then at least 30 minutes off.

4. If help may be delayed or if the child is to be transported, use a splint to keep the area immobilized (see later section on splints).

Additional Care

- Treat the child for shock.
- Monitor the child's breathing.
- Remove clothing and jewelry if they may cut off circulation as swelling occurs.

ALERT

Dislocation

Do not try to put the displaced bone back in place. Do not let the child eat or drink.

Sprains

Sprains can range from mild to severe. It may be difficult to tell a severe sprain from a fracture, but the first aid is similar for both. The ankles, knees, wrists, and fingers are the body parts most often sprained.

When You See

- Signs of pain
- Swollen joint
- Bruising of joint area
- Inability to use joint

Do This First

1. Have the child rest. Immobilize the injured area in the position in which you find it.
2. Put ice or a cold pack on the area and then wrap joint with a compression bandage. Remove the cold pack after 20 minutes, for at least 30 minutes.
3. Use a soft splint (bandage, pillow, blanket) to immobilize and support the joint.
4. Elevate a sprained hand or ankle above the level of the heart (Figure 7-3).
5. Seek medical attention.

Additional Care

- Remove clothing or jewelry if they may cut off circulation as swelling occurs.

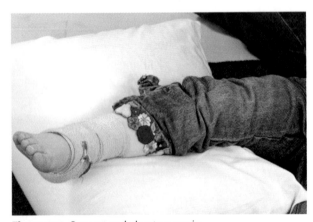

Figure 7-3 Support and elevate a sprain.

MUSCLE INJURIES

Common muscle injuries include strains, contusions, and cramps. These injuries are usually less serious than bone and joint injuries.

Strains

A **strain** is a tearing of the muscle caused by overexerting or "pulling" a muscle. Strains are common sports injuries.

When You See

- Signs of dull or sharp pain when muscle is used
- Stiffness of the area
- Weakness or inability to use the muscle normally

Do This First

1. Rest the muscle.
2. Put ice or a cold pack on the area: 20 minutes on, then at least 30 minutes off.
3. With an extremity, wrap a compression bandage around the muscle.
4. Elevate the limb.

Additional Care

- Seek medical attention if pain is severe or persists.

Contusions

A **contusion** is a bruised muscle as may result from a blow.

When You See

- Signs of pain
- Swollen, tender area
- Skin discoloration (black and blue)

Do This First

1. Rest the muscle.
2. Put ice or a cold pack on the area: 20 minutes on, then at least 30 minutes off for the first 2 to 3 hours.

3. With an extremity, wrap a compression bandage around the muscle.

4. Elevate the limb.

Additional Care

- Seek medical attention if pain is severe or persists.

Cramps

A muscle cramp is a tightening of a muscle usually caused by prolonged use. Cramps are common in the legs, stomach, back, or any muscle that is overused. These cramps are different from heat cramps, which result from fluid loss in hot environments (see Chapter 10).

When You See

- Signs of muscle pain and tightness

Do This First

1. Gently stretch out the muscle if possible.
2. Allow the child to gently massage the muscle if this provides relief.

Additional Care

- Have the child drink plenty of fluids.

RICE

The RICE acronym is an easy way to remember how to treat all bone, joint, and muscle injuries. With this procedure you do not have to know whether the injury is a fracture, dislocation, sprain, or strain, because they are treated in the same manner.

R = Rest

I = Ice

C = Compression

E = Elevation

Rest

Any movement of a musculoskeletal injury can cause further injury, pain, and swelling. Have the child rest until medical help arrives. Rest is also important for healing.

Ice

Cold reduces swelling, lessens pain, and minimizes bruising. Put ice or a cold pack on the injury (except for an open fracture) as soon as possible. Cubed or crushed ice in a plastic bag, or an improvised cold pack such as a bag of frozen peas or a cloth pad soaked in cold water (refreshed with cold water every 10 minutes), can be applied on top of a thin cloth placed directly on the injured area. A commercial cold pack should be wrapped in cloth to prevent direct skin contact because it may be cold enough to freeze the skin.

Cold works best if applied to the injury as soon as possible, preferably within 10 minutes. Apply it for 20 minutes on and at least 30 minutes off for the first few hours, then for 20 minutes at a time every 2 or 3 hours for the first 24 to 48 hours, or for 72 hours for severe injuries.

Compression

Compression of an injured extremity is done with an elastic roller bandage. Compression may help prevent internal bleeding and swelling. Wrap the bandage over the injured area. It can also be used around a cold pack. Check the child's fingers or toes frequently to make sure circulation is not cut off.

Elevation

Elevating an injured arm or leg also may help prevent swelling and control internal or external bleeding. Splint a fracture first, and elevate it only if moving the limb does not cause pain.

SPLINTING THE EXTREMITIES

In most childcare centers, splinting is seldom used because medical help will arrive soon and because moving the injured area to apply the splint may cause additional damage. In these cases it is generally recommended to help prevent movement of the injured area with pillows or other thick, soft padding.

In some other situations, however, when a child has a fracture, dislocation, or sprain in

Perform the Skill

RICE

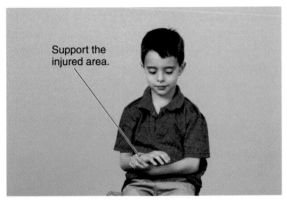

Support the injured area.

1 Rest the injured area.

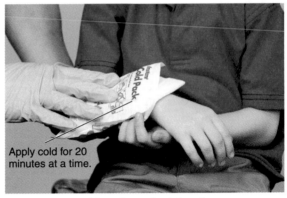

Apply cold for 20 minutes at a time.

2 Put ice or cold pack on the injured area.

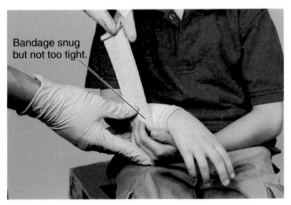

Bandage snug but not too tight.

3 Compress the injured area with an elastic roller bandage.

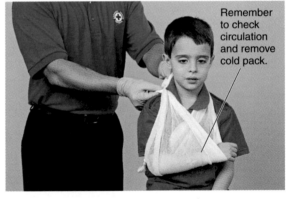

Remember to check circulation and remove cold pack.

4 Elevate the injured area using a sling.

an arm or leg, the arm or leg may be splinted if the child is at risk for moving the injured area—unless help is expected within a few minutes. Always splint an extremity before transporting a child to a healthcare provider or emergency department. Splinting helps prevent further injury, reduces pain, and minimizes bleeding and swelling.

Types of Splints and Slings

Splints can be made from many different materials at hand (**Figure 7-4**). There are three types of splints:

- **Rigid splints** may be made from a board, a piece of plastic or metal, a rolled newspaper or magazine, or thick cardboard.
- **Soft splints** may be made from a pillow, folded blanket or towel, or a triangular bandage folded into a sling.
- **Anatomic splints** involve splinting an injured leg to the uninjured leg or splinting fingers together.

Splints can be tied in place with bandages, belts, neckties, or strips of cloth torn from clothing.

Guidelines for Splinting

- Put a dressing on any open wound before splinting the area.
- Splint only if it does not cause more pain for the child.
- Splint the injury in the position you find it (**Figure 7-5**).
- Splint to immobilize the entire area. With an extremity, splint the joints above and below the injured area.
- Put padding such as cloth between the splint and the skin.

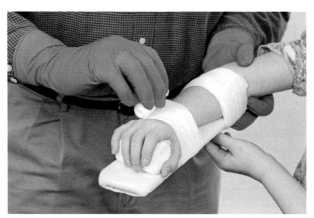

(a) Rigid splint.

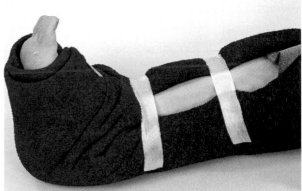

(b) Soft splint.

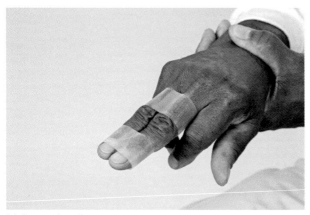

(c) Anatomic splint.

Figure 7-4 Examples of splints.

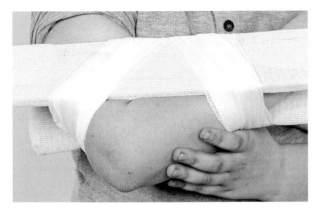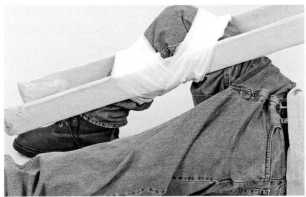

Figure 7-5 Splint an injury in the position found, such as these elbow and knee injuries. Do not try to straighten the limb to splint it.

- Put splints on both sides of a fractured bone if possible.
- Elevate the splinted extremity if possible.
- Apply ice or a cold pack to the injury around the splint.
- With a splinted extremity, check the child's fingers or toes frequently to make sure circulation is not cut off. Swelling, bluish discoloration, tingling or numbness, and cold skin are signs and symptoms of reduced circulation. If any of these are noted, the splint should be removed.

Follow the steps shown in the Perform the Skill examples to splint an arm or leg. After splinting an arm, secure with a sling and binder. A sling supports and elevates an injury of the hand or forearm. A sling may also be used to minimize movement and support the area with a shoulder dislocation or rib fracture. A leg fracture can be splinted using either a rigid splint or an anatomic splint (as shown in the example). The example shows splinting of a lower leg fracture. A similar splint can be used for an upper leg fracture, with the bandages tied higher (including the hips).

Perform the Skill

Splinting an Arm

Support above and below the injury.

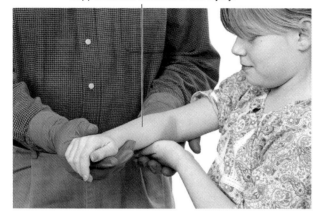

1 Support the arm.

If available, add
a roller bandage.   Pad the splint.

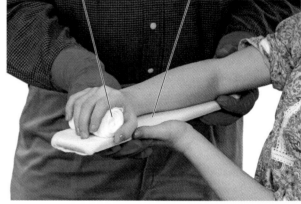

2 Position the arm on a rigid splint.

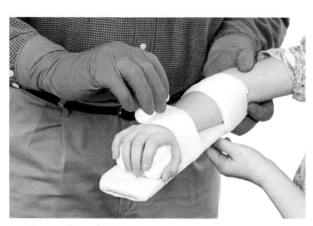

3 Secure the splint.

Check for tingling or numbness, swelling or cold skin.

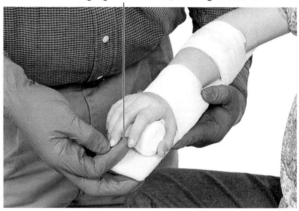

4 Check circulation.

Perform the Skill

Making an Arm Sling and Binder

Use a safety pin or tie the point at the elbow.

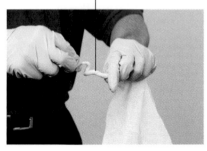

1 Secure the point of the bandage at the elbow.

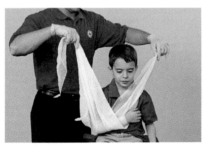

2 Position the triangular bandage.

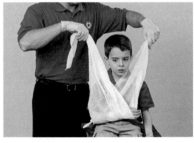

3 Bring up the lower end of the bandage to the opposite side of the neck.

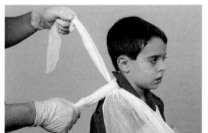

4 Tie the ends.

Pad under the knot.

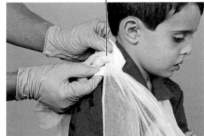

5 Pad the knot.

A binder helps prevent movement.

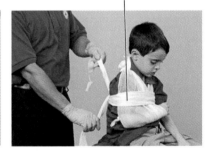

6 Tie a binder bandage over the sling and around the chest.

Perform the Skill

Splinting a Leg

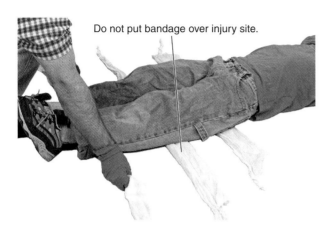

Do not put bandage over injury site.

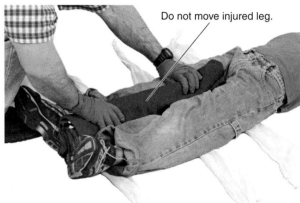

Do not move injured leg.

1 Gently slide 2 or 3 bandages or strips of cloth under both legs.

2 Put padding between the legs.

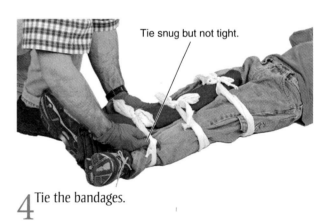

Tie snug but not tight.

3 Gently slide the uninjured leg next to the injured leg.

4 Tie the bandages.

8 Sudden Illness

The illnesses described in this chapter may occur in children suddenly or without much warning that the child is becoming ill. In many cases the child's condition can rapidly become serious or life threatening, and you need to act quickly. In a childcare center, follow the center's policy for when to take action in an emergency and when to call the child's parents for less urgent medical care.

The following sections describe sudden illnesses that may affect children. You do not have to know for sure what the child's specific illness is, however, before you give first aid.

General signs and symptoms of sudden illness:

- Child feels ill, dizzy, confused, or weak
- Skin color changes (flushed or pale), sweating
- Nausea, vomiting

General care for sudden illness:

1. Call 9-1-1 for unexplained sudden illness.
2. Help the child rest and avoid getting chilled or overheated.
3. Reassure the child.
4. Do not give the child anything to eat or drink.
5. Watch for changes, and be prepared to give basic life support (BLS).

MENINGITIS

Meningitis is an inflammation of the meninges, the covering of the brain and spinal cord. It is a rare but life-threatening emergency. This disease is contagious and usually occurs in outbreaks. The signs and symptoms often come on quickly.

When You See

- Fever
- Chills
- Nausea, vomiting, loss of appetite

- Stiff neck
- Headache
- Convulsions
- Sensitivity to light

Do This First

1. If you suspect meningitis, or the child has been exposed to meningitis, call 9-1-1 or a healthcare provider immediately.
2. Keep the child comfortable and resting until seen by a healthcare provider.

Additional Care

- Keep other children away from a child suspected of having meningitis.

DEHYDRATION

Dehydration occurs when the child loses significant amounts of body fluids, as may occur with heat exhaustion (see Chapter 10), diarrhea, or vomiting. Dehydration in infants and young children can be a serious condition.

When You See

- Sunken eyes
- Listlessness
- Dry mouth
- Infrequent urination and concentrated urine

Do This First

1. Give frequent drinks of clear fluids.
2. Seek medical attention if the infant or child will not drink or has repeated vomiting or diarrhea.

NEAR DROWNING

Infants and small children can drown quickly in a bath or pool. **Near drowning** is a condition that occurs when the child has been under water a prolonged time but may still be resuscitated. Note that children immersed in cold water have been successfully resuscitated after a lengthy time.

When You See

- An unresponsive child in water

Do This First

1. Remove the child from water, carrying the child with head lower than chest.
2. Have someone call 9-1-1 immediately. Check for breathing. If you are alone and the child needs CPR (see Chapter 2), give help for 2 minutes, then call 9-1-1 if it was not already called. Then continue BLS.
3. Be prepared for vomiting and to turn the child on his or her side.
4. If the child has signs of circulation and is breathing, place him or her in the recovery position.

Additional Care

- Call 9-1-1 even if the child recovers, because water in the lungs may still cause damage.

ASTHMA

Asthma is a common problem affecting one in seven children. In an asthma attack the airway becomes narrow and the child has difficulty breathing. Most children with asthma you will encounter in a childcare setting have already been diagnosed and will have prescribed medication for emergency situations. You should be prepared to help the child with this medication following your childcare center's policy (**Figure 8-1**). Untreated, a severe asthma attack can be fatal.

Asthma Triggers

Asthma attacks are usually triggered by some factor in the child's internal or external environment. Understanding these factors helps prevent or minimize a child's attacks. Common triggers include:

- Respiratory infection, including the common cold (most common cause in children under age 5)

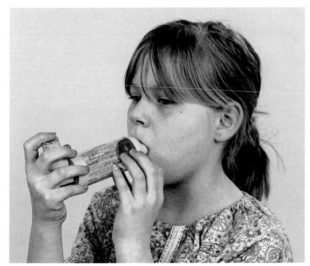

Figure 8-1 Many children with asthma use an inhaler with a spacer.

- Allergic reaction to pollen, mold, dust mites, animal fur or dander
- Exercise (especially in cold, dry air)
- Certain foods (nuts, eggs, milk)
- Emotional stress
- Medications
- Air pollution caused by such things as cigarette smoke, vehicle exhaust, or fumes of cleaning products
- Temperature extremes

Knowing the specific triggers that provoke a child's asthma can help you prevent attacks. The child may have had a skin test to detect specific allergens that trigger his or her asthma. In addition to keeping the child away from the factors listed above, follow these guidelines:

- Use a damp cloth to dust furniture and surfaces.
- Vacuum rugs frequently (when the child is not present).
- Avoid fluffy blankets and pillows that collect dust and those that contain feathers.
- Enclose mattress and pillow in plastic covers.
- Do not use air fresheners or products with strong odors.
- Use an air purifier and keep child indoors when pollen counts are high.

The Child's Treatment Plan

When a child has been diagnosed with asthma, the healthcare provider should provide a detailed management plan. A childcare center should have a copy of this plan. It should include:

- Activities and triggers to avoid
- How to treat the child's asthma
- Prescribed medications and when and how to use them
- What to do and who to call in an emergency

Know where this plan and the child's medications are kept and what to do if an asthma or other breathing emergency occurs. Note that in some states, childcare providers are required to have specific information on the use of inhaled medications.

When You See
- Wheezing and difficulty breathing and speaking
- Dry, persistent cough
- Fear, anxiety, fatigue, restlessness
- Gray-blue skin
- Changing levels of responsiveness

Do This First
1. If the child is not known to have asthma (first attack), call 9-1-1 immediately.
2. If the child is known to have asthma, help the child use his or her medication (usually an inhaler).
3. Help the child rest and sit in a position for easiest breathing.
4. The child may use the inhaler again in 5 to 10 minutes if needed (follow specific instructions for this child).

Additional Care
- If the breathing difficulty persists after using the inhaler, call 9-1-1.

Using a Peak Flow Meter

A **peak flow meter** is a device used to monitor the child's breathing ability—it is not used when an asthma attack occurs. The child's treatment plan may call for use of the peak flow meter at routine times and recording or charting the results. The meter is used this way:

1. The child takes a full breath in.
2. The child seals his or her lips around the mouthpiece and exhales out as hard and fast as possible.
3. The reading is taken from the position of the pointer on the meter.

How to Use a Metered-Dose Inhaler

Always follow the healthcare provider's specific instructions for helping a child use his or her inhaler, a device that contains and delivers the asthma medication. Following are general instructions that may need to be modified for the specific medication device or a particular child.

1. Shake the inhaler.
2. If a spacer is used, position it on the inhaler. (A spacer is a tube or chamber that fits between the inhaler and the child's mouth.)
3. Have the child breathe out fully through the mouth.
4. With the child's lips around the inhaler mouthpiece or the spacer, have the child inhale slowly and deeply; press the inhaler down to release one spray of medication as the child inhales. (A facemask is generally used for an infant instead of a mouthpiece.)
5. Have the child hold his or her breath for up to 10 seconds if possible and then exhale slowly. Follow the directions for the inhaler or the child's treatment plan to repeat doses if needed.

How to Use a Nebulizer

Some children use a nebulizer rather than an inhaler to administer their asthma medication. A **nebulizer** uses an air compressor to make a fine mist of the medication for the child to breathe. Nebulizer equipment includes a compressor with tubing to a nebulizer cup attached to a mouthpiece or face mask (**Figure 8-2**). As with

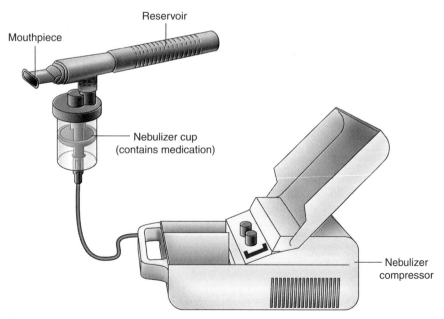

Figure 8-2 Parts of a nebulizer.

an inhaler, follow the specific instructions from the equipment manufacturer and healthcare provider. Following are the general instructions that may need to be modified for the specific device or a particular child.

1. Have the child sit in a quiet place away from other children.
2. Assemble the equipment.
3. Measure the medication and place it in the nebulizer cup.
4. Plug in the compressor and turn it on.
5. Using either the mouthpiece or mask, have the child breathe slowly and deeply until the medication cup is empty (**Figure 8-3**).

The nebulizer equipment should be cleaned after each use, following the equipment manufacturer's instructions. Generally, you take the pieces apart, wash the plastic pieces with soap and water, and let them dry. Note that lemon-scented or other strongly perfumed soap should not be used to wash this equipment because a perfumed soap can be irritating to someone with lung disease. The compressor may be wiped clean. The air filter on the compressor is periodically replaced. Store the unit in its container.

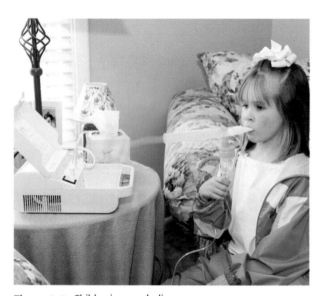

Figure 8-3 Child using a nebulizer.

CROUP

Croup is an inflammation of the airway caused by a viral infection and is common in children between 3 months and 5 years of age. The symptoms are usually mild, but severe breathing difficulty requires medical attention.

When You See
- Barking cough
- Harsh noisy breathing (especially when inhaling)
- Use of head, neck, and abdominal muscles in breathing
- With breathing difficulty: bluish color of tongue and lips

Do This First
1. For severe breathing difficulty, seek immediate medical attention.
2. Help child sit up comfortably, or hold a small child, in position for easiest breathing.
3. Use a cool mist or steam vaporizer, and have the child breathe in the moist air. (If a vaporizer is not available, steam up the bathroom by running a hot shower.)

Additional Care
- If the attack of croup lasts longer than 15 minutes or seems severe, seek medical attention.
- If the child has not recovered from the viral infection within a few days, a healthcare provider should be seen.

ALERT

Steam Vaporizer
If the vaporizer produces hot steam, do not let child get too close to it.

HYPERVENTILATION

Hyperventilation is fast, deep breathing caused by anxiety or stress.

When You See

- Very fast breathing rate
- Dizziness, faintness
- Tingling or numbness in hands and feet
- Muscle twitching or cramping

Do This First

1. Make sure there is no other cause for the breathing difficulty to care for.
2. Reassure the child and ask him or her to try to breathe slowly.
3. Call 9-1-1 if the child's breathing does not return to normal within a few minutes.

Additional Care

- A child who often has this problem should see a healthcare provider, because some medical conditions can cause rapid breathing.

RESPIRATORY DISTRESS

Respiratory distress, or difficulty breathing, can be caused by many different illnesses and injuries. If you can know the cause of a child's breathing difficulty, such as asthma or croup (described earlier), give first aid for that problem. Otherwise, give this general breathing care.

When You See

- Child is gasping or unable to catch his or her breath
- Breathing is faster or slower, or deeper or shallower, than normal
- Breathing involves sounds such as wheezing or gurgling
- Child feels dizzy or lightheaded

Do This First

1. Call 9-1-1 for sudden unexplained breathing problems.
2. Help the child rest in position of easiest breathing.
3. If you have a prescribed medicine for the child, follow your childcare center's policy to help the child take it if needed.
4. Stay with the child and be prepared to give BLS.

Additional Care

- Calm and reassure the child (anxiety increases breathing distress).

FAINTING

Fainting is caused by a temporary reduced blood flow to the brain. This commonly occurs in hot weather or after a prolonged period of inactivity, or from other causes such as pain, fright, or lack of food. If a child seems about to faint (feeling weak and dizzy, with a very pale face), have the child lie down with legs raised 8 to 12 inches (**Figure 8-4**).

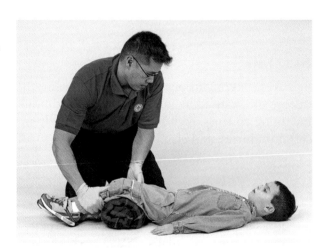

Figure 8-4 Position for a child about to faint.

When You See

- Sudden brief loss of responsiveness and collapse
- Pale, cool skin, sweating

Do This First

1. Check the child's breathing and provide BLS if needed.
2. Lay the child down and raise the legs 8 to 12 inches. Loosen any tight clothing.
3. Check for possible injuries caused by falling.
4. Reassure the child as he or she recovers.

Additional Care

- Call 9-1-1 if the child does not regain responsiveness soon or faints repeatedly.
- Place an unresponsive child who is breathing in the recovery position to let the mouth drain in case of vomiting.

ALERT

Fainting

Do not give a child who feels faint anything to drink.

SEIZURES

Seizures, or convulsions, result from a brain disturbance caused by many different conditions, including epilepsy, high fever in young children, certain injuries, and electric shock.

When You See

- *Minor seizures:* staring blankly ahead; slight twitching of lips, head, or arms and legs; other movements such as lip-smacking or chewing
- *Major seizures:* crying out and then becoming unresponsive; body becomes rigid and then shakes in convulsions; jaw may clench

- *Fever convulsions in young children:* hot, flushed skin; violent muscle twitching; arched back; clenched fists

Do This First

1. Try to catch a child who is about to fall. Prevent injury during the seizure by moving away dangerous objects and putting something flat and soft (or your hand) under the child's head (**Figure 8-5**).
2. Loosen clothing around the neck to ease breathing.
3. Gently turn the child onto one side to help keep the airway clear if vomiting occurs.
4. Monitor the child's breathing and give BLS if needed.
5. Be reassuring as the child regains responsiveness.

Additional Care

- Call 9-1-1 if the seizure lasts more than 5 minutes, if the child is not known to have epilepsy, if the child does not recover within 10 minutes, if the child has trouble breathing or has another seizure, if the child is known to have another medical condition, or if the child is injured.
- For an infant or child with fever convulsions, sponge the body with room temperature water to help cool the body, and call 9-1-1.

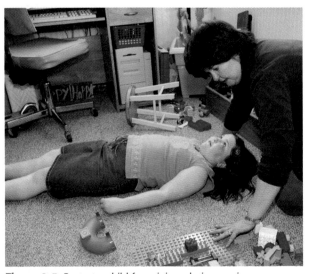

Figure 8-5 Protect a child from injury during a seizure.

Fever Convulsions

Younger children (generally between six months and four years of age) may have a seizure because of a rapidly rising fever. These are sometimes called **febrile seizures.** Give the same care for the seizure as described earlier, and then try to cool the child's body. Remove clothing and sponge the child's body with room temperature water; do not let the child get cold. Seek urgent medical attention.

SEVERE ABDOMINAL PAIN

Abdominal injuries are described in Chapter 6; always call 9-1-1 for an abdominal injury. Abdominal pain may also result from illness ranging from minor conditions to serious medical emergencies. Urgent medical care is needed for any severe abdominal pain in these situations:

- Sudden, severe, intolerable pain, or pain that causes awakening from sleep
- Pain that begins in the general area of the central abdomen and later moves to the lower right
- Pain with a swollen abdomen that feels hard
- Pain with a hard lump in lower abdomen or groin area
- Pain accompanied by difficulty breathing
- Pain that occurs suddenly, stops, and then returns without warning
- Pain accompanied by red or purple, jelly-like stool; or with blood or mucus in stool
- Pain accompanied by greenish-brown vomit

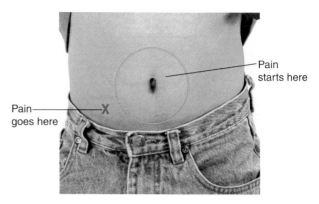

Figure 8-6 Locations of appendicitis pain.

Appendicitis

Appendicitis, or inflammation of the appendix, may occur in a child of any age. Waves of pain begin in the middle of the abdomen and settle in severe pain in the right lower abdomen, along with fever, nausea with or without vomiting or diarrhea, and loss of appetite (**Figure 8-6**). Have the child lie down, and call 9-1-1 immediately. Do not give the child anything to eat or drink.

DIABETIC EMERGENCIES

Children with diabetes generally require daily insulin injections. Their meals and activity levels must also be regulated to maintain a balance of blood sugar and insulin in the body. Childcare providers should be aware of a child's diabetes and have received instructions from the parents on managing this condition and problems that may occur. Low blood sugar is called **hypoglycemia,** and high blood sugar is called **hyperglycemia.** Many factors can cause either of these conditions, which are more common in children with undiagnosed or newly diagnosed diabetes. Hypoglycemia is more common and often occurs quickly. Either condition can quickly progress to a medical emergency if the child is not treated.

Low Blood Sugar

When You See

- Sudden dizziness, weakness, shakiness, or mood change (irritability or combativeness)
- Headache, confusion, difficulty paying attention
- Pale skin, sweating
- Hunger
- Clumsy, jerky movements
- Possible seizure

Do This First

1. Confirm that the child is known to have diabetes; look for a medical ID. Follow your childcare center's instructions for how much sugar to give the child.
2. Give a fully responsive child sugar: glucose tablets, fruit juice, sugar packets (but *not* non-sugar sweetener packets), or hard candy (unless choking is a risk) **(Figure 8-7)**.
3. Call 9-1-1 immediately so that EMS personnel can assess the child and provide additional treatment as needed.
4. If after 15 minutes EMS has not responded and the child still feels ill or has signs and symptoms, give more sugar.

Additional Care

- If the child becomes unresponsive or continues to have significant signs and symptoms, monitor the child's breathing and provide BLS while waiting for help.

ALERT

Diabetic Emergency Alert!
If a diabetic child becomes unresponsive, do not try to inject insulin or put food or fluids in the mouth.

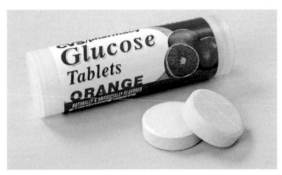

Figure 8-7 Glucose tablets.

High Blood Sugar

When You See

- Frequent urination
- Drowsiness
- Dry mouth, thirst
- Shortness of breath, deep rapid breathing
- Breath smells fruity
- Nausea, vomiting
- Eventual unresponsiveness

Do This First

1. Confirm that the child has diabetes; look for a medical ID.
2. Follow the child's healthcare provider's instructions for hyperglycemia.
3. If you cannot judge whether the child has low or high blood sugar, give sugar as for low blood sugar. Call 9-1-1.
4. Call 9-1-1 if the child becomes unresponsive or continues to have significant signs and symptoms.

Additional Care

- Put an unresponsive child who is breathing in the recovery position and monitor breathing.

9 Poisoning

Poisoning is a common emergency in young children.

SWALLOWED POISONS

Many substances in home and childcare settings are poisonous if swallowed.

When You See

- Open container of poisonous substance
- A burn or smell around the child's mouth
- Nausea, vomiting, abdominal cramps
- Drowsiness, dizziness, disorientation
- Changing levels of responsiveness

Do This First

1. Clean any remaining poison from the child's mouth, and remove any contaminated clothing.
2. Determine what was swallowed, when, and how much.
3. *For a responsive child,* call the national Poison Control Center (1-800-222-1222) immediately and follow their instructions.
4. *For an unresponsive child,* call 9-1-1 and provide basic life support (BLS) as needed.

Additional Care

- Put an unresponsive child who is breathing in the recovery position and be prepared for vomiting.
- If a responsive child's mouth or lips are burned by a corrosive chemical, rinse the mouth with cold water (without swallowing).

ALERT

Swallowed Poison

Do not give activated charcoal or any other substance unless told to do so by the Poison Control Center.

Food Poisoning

Food poisoning signs and symptoms may begin soon after eating or within a day.

When You See

- Nausea and vomiting, signs of abdominal pain or cramps
- Diarrhea, possibly with blood
- Headache, fever

Do This First

1. Have the child rest lying down.
2. Give the child fluids to drink.
3. Seek medical attention.

Additional Care

- Talk with the child's parents, who should check with others with whom the child has eaten recently.

ALERT

Botulism

Botulism is more likely from home-canned foods. If the child experiences dizziness, muscle weakness, and difficulty talking or breathing, call 9-1-1.

PREVENTING FOOD POISONING

To prevent food poisoning:
- Fully defrost frozen poultry and meat before cooking.
- Fully cook poultry, meat, fish, and eggs to kill bacteria.
- Do not keep cooked foods lukewarm a long time before serving.
- Wash hands before preparing food; wash anytime after touching uncooked poultry.

Poisonous Plants

If a child eats a part of a plant, unless you are absolutely certain the plant is nonpoisonous, call the Poison Control Center and give first aid as for swallowed poisons. Remove any plant parts remaining in the child's mouth. Take a piece of the plant with you to the telephone to help you describe it (**Figure 9-1**).

Alcohol

Even a small amount of alcohol consumed by a child, including the alcohol in many cough syrups, can lead to a medical emergency.

When You See

- Smell of alcohol about the child
- Flushed, moist face
- Slurred speech, staggering
- Nausea
- Changing levels of responsiveness

Do This First

1. Check for injuries or illness. Note that a child with uncontrolled diabetes may appear to be intoxicated.

2. *For a responsive intoxicated child:*
   a. Stay with the child and protect him or her from injury.
   b. Do not let the child lie down on his or her back.

3. *For an unresponsive intoxicated child:*
   a. If the child is breathing, position the child in the recovery position, preferably on the left side.
   b. Monitor the child's breathing and provide BLS if necessary.
   c. Call 9-1-1 if the child's breathing is irregular, if seizures occur, or if the child cannot be roused (coma).

Drug Abuse or Overdose

A child under the influence of any drug or prescription medication may have a wide range of behaviors and symptoms, depending on the specific drug. In some cases it is impossible to know whether behavior or symptoms are caused by a drug or by an injury or sudden illness. Follow these general guidelines.

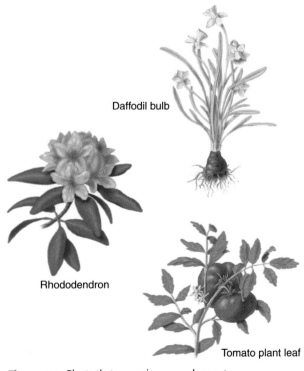

Daffodil bulb

Rhododendron

Tomato plant leaf

Figure 9-1 Plants that are poisonous when eaten.

When You See

- Very small or large pupils of the eye (see Figure 6-1)
- Stumbling, clumsiness, drowsiness, incoherent speech
- Difficulty breathing (very slow or fast)
- Irrational or violent behavior
- Changing levels of responsiveness
- Evidence of a suicide attempt

Do This First

1. Put an *unresponsive child* who is breathing in the recovery position, preferably on the left side, and give BLS as needed. Call 9-1-1.
2. For a *responsive child,* try to find out what drug the child took. If there is evidence of an overdose, call 9-1-1.
3. If symptoms are minor and you know the substance taken, call the Poison Control Center and follow their instructions.

Additional Care

- Monitor the child's condition while waiting for help.
- Provide care for any condition that occurs (seizures, shock, cardiac arrest).

INHALED POISONS

Various gases and fumes may be present in different settings. Unless you know the specific treatment for inhaling a gas, care for a child with a suspected gas inhalation the same as for carbon monoxide.

Carbon Monoxide

Carbon monoxide is especially dangerous because it is invisible, odorless, and tasteless—and very lethal. Carbon monoxide may be present from motor vehicle exhaust, a faulty furnace or other heater, a fireplace or stove, or fire. Exposure to large amounts causes an immediate poisoning reaction. A slow or small leak may cause gradual poisoning with less dramatic symptoms. To prevent poisoning, carbon monoxide detectors should be used along with smoke detectors in appropriate locations.

When You See

- Headache
- Dizziness, lightheadedness, confusion, weakness
- Nausea, vomiting
- Signs of chest pain
- Convulsions
- Changing levels of responsiveness

Do This First

1. Immediately move the child into fresh air.
2. Call 9-1-1 even if the child starts to recover.
3. Monitor the child's breathing and give BLS as needed.

Additional Care

- Put an unresponsive child who is breathing in the recovery position.
- Loosen tight clothing around the neck or chest.

POISON IVY, OAK, AND SUMAC

Contact with poison ivy, oak, and sumac plants causes an allergic skin reaction in about half of all children (Figure 9-2). Once the rash appears on the skin and has been washed, however, it cannot spread to anyone else. It is not a contagious condition but a reaction to a substance in the plant. It may take up to two weeks for the rash to heal.

When You See

- Redness and extreme itching occurring first
- Rash, blisters (may weep)
- Possible headache and fever

Do This First

1. Wash the area thoroughly with soap and water as soon as possible after contact.
2. For severe reactions or swelling on the face or groin area, the child needs medical attention.
3. Follow your childcare center's policy to treat itching with colloid oatmeal baths; a paste made of baking soda and water, calamine lotion, or topical

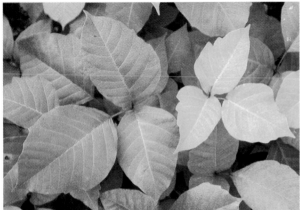

(a) Poison ivy

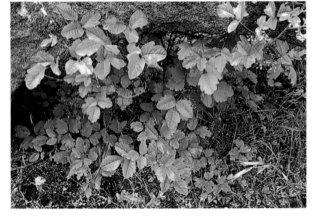

(b) Poison oak

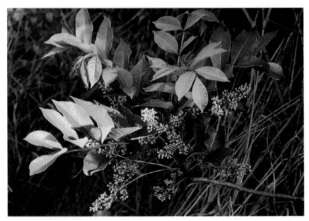

(c) Poison sumac

Figure 9-2 Poisonous plants.

hydrocortisone cream; and an oral antihistamine. Parental permission is required.

Additional Care

- Wash clothing and shoes (and pets) that contacted the plants to prevent further spread.
- Childcare providers should inform the child's parents of an exposure to a poisonous plant, which may produce a rash hours or days later.

ALERT

Poison Ivy/Oak/Sumac

Do not burn these poisonous plants to get rid of them as smoke also spreads the poisonous substance.

BITES AND STINGS

Animal Bites

Animal bites cause a wound and carry the risk of rabies, which can be fatal without prompt treatment. Rabies should be suspected in cases of unprovoked attacks, strangely acting animals, or wild (nondomestic) animals.

When You See

- Any animal bite

Do This First

1. Wearing medical exam gloves, clean the wound with soap and water. Run water over the wound for 5 minutes (except for large wounds or severe bleeding).
2. Control the bleeding.
3. Cover the wound with a sterile dressing and bandage (see Chapter 3).
4. The child should see a healthcare provider or go to the emergency department right away. Follow your childcare center's policy.

Additional Care

- All animal bites must be reported to local animal control officers or police. The law requires certain procedures to be followed when rabies is a risk.
- Check that the child's tetanus vaccination is up to date (see Chapter 3).

ALERT

Animal Bite

Do not try to catch any animal that may have rabies.

Human Bites

Because our mouths are full of germs, if a child is bitten by another child and the skin is broken, a wound infection may result.

When You See

- A human bite
- Open puncture wound
- Bleeding

Do This First

1. Wearing medical exam gloves, clean the wound with soap and water. Run water over wound for 5 minutes (except when bleeding severely).
2. Control bleeding.
3. Cover the wound with a sterile dressing and bandage (see Chapter 3).
4. The child should be seen by a healthcare provider or go to the emergency department right away. Follow your childcare center's policy.

Additional Care

- If any tissue has been bitten off, it should be taken with the child to the emergency department.
- Check that the child's tetanus vaccination is up to date (see Chapter 3).

Snakebites

Poisonous snakes in North America include rattlesnakes, copperheads, water moccasins (cottonmouths), coral snakes, and exotic species kept in captivity. Rattlesnake bites cause most snakebite deaths. Treat all snakebites in children as potentially dangerous. Antivenin is often available in areas where snakebites are common. See Chapter 16 on preventing snakebites when children are outdoors.

When You See

- Puncture marks in skin
- Complaint of pain or burning at bite site
- Redness and swelling
- *Depending on snake species:* difficulty breathing, numbness or muscle paralysis, nausea and vomiting, blurred vision, drowsiness or confusion, weakness

Do This First

1. Have the child lie down and stay calm. (Do not move the child unless absolutely necessary.) Keep the bitten area immobile and below the level of the heart.
2. Call 9-1-1.
3. Wash the bite wound with soap and water.
4. Remove jewelry or tight clothing before swelling begins.

Additional Care

- Do not try to catch the snake, but note its appearance and describe it to the healthcare provider.
- Stay with the child, monitor his or her breathing, and give BLS if needed.

ALERT

Snakebite

Do not put a tourniquet on a snakebite.

Pit Vipers

According to the Wilderness Medical Society, a child bitten by a pit viper, such as rattlesnake, may have one or two puncture wounds about ½-inch apart. Swelling can occur rapidly and involve the entire extremity. The child may become nauseated, vomit, sweat, and complain of weakness. Care involves removing the child and any bystanders from the snake. If possible, attempt to identify the snake's markings from a safe distance. Minimize movement of the child. Seek immediate medical attention. Gently wash the area with soap and water if available.

Coral Snakes

For snakebites from coral snakes only, a bitten extremity should be wrapped snugly but not tightly with an elastic bandage. You should be able to insert one finger under the bandage. Wrap the entire length of the extremity to reduce the spread of the venom by slowing lymph flow. The extremity should also be immobilized, and the victim should receive medical attention as soon as possible.

Spider Bites

Many types of spiders bite, but only the venom of the black widow and brown recluse spider is serious and sometimes fatal (**Figure 9-3**). The black widow often has a red hourglass-shaped marking on the underside of the abdomen. The brown recluse has a violin-shaped marking on its back. An antivenin is available for black widow spider bites.

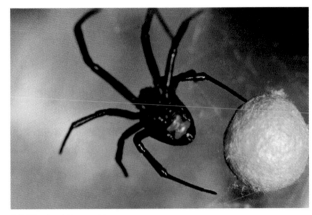

(a) Black widow spider

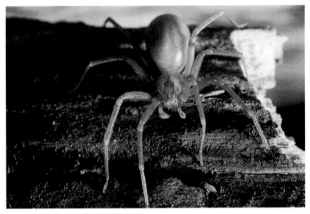

(b) Brown recluse spider

Figure 9-3 Poisonous spiders.

When You See

For black widow bite:

- Complaint of pain at bite site
- Red skin at site
- After 15 minutes to hours: sweating, nausea, stomach and muscle cramps, increased pain at site, dizziness or weakness, difficulty breathing

For brown recluse bite:

- Stinging sensation at site
- Over 8 to 48 hours: increasing pain, blistering at site, fever, chills, nausea or vomiting, joint pain, open sore at site

Do This First

1. If the child has difficulty breathing, call 9-1-1 and be prepared to give BLS. Call 9-1-1 immediately for a brown recluse spider bite.
2. Keep the bite area below the level of the heart.
3. Wash the area with soap and water.
4. Put ice or a cold pack on the bite area.

Additional Care

- Try to safely catch the spider to show it to the healthcare provider.
- If 9-1-1 was not called, the child needs to be taken to the emergency department.

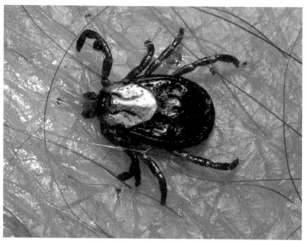

(a) Tick embedded in skin

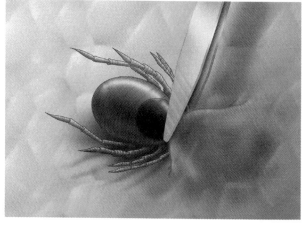

Figure 9-5 Grasp tick close to the skin and pull very gently.

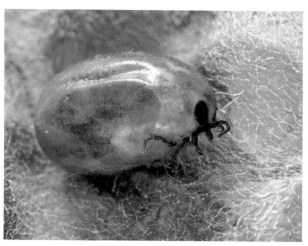

(b) Tick engorged

Figure 9-4 Tick bite.

Tick Bites

Tick bites are not poisonous but can transmit serious diseases like Rocky Mountain spotted fever or Lyme disease. The tick embeds its mouth parts in the skin and may remain for days (**Figure 9-4**).

When You See

- Tick embedded in skin

Do This First

1. Remove the tick by grasping it close to the skin with tweezers and pulling very gently until the tick finally lets go. Avoid pulling too hard or jerking, which may leave part of the tick in the skin (**Figure 9-5**).
2. Wash the area with soap and water.
3. Follow your childcare center's policy to put an antiseptic, such as rubbing alcohol, on the site followed by an antibiotic cream.

Additional Care

- Seek medical attention if a rash appears around the site or the child later experiences fever, chills, joint pain, or other flu-like symptoms.

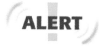

ALERT

Tick Removal

Do not try to remove an embedded tick by covering it with petroleum jelly, soaking it with bleach, burning it away with a hot pin or other object, or similar methods. These methods may result in part of the tick remaining embedded in the skin.

LYME DISEASE

Lyme disease, spread by ticks, has become a serious problem in many areas in the United States. Lyme disease is a bacterial infectious

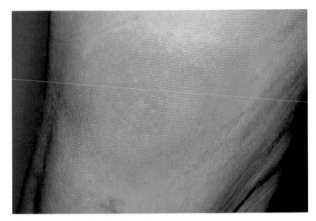

Figure 9-6 Lyme disease bull's-eye rash.

disease that first causes fever, chills, and other flu-like symptoms and later on may cause heart and neurological problems. Look for a bull's-eye rash that appears around the tick bite site 3 to 30 days later. If this rash, flu-like symptoms, or joint pain occurs after a tick bite, the child needs medical attention (**Figure 9-6**).

Bee and Wasp Stings

Bee, wasp, and other insect stings are common in children playing outdoors. These stings are not poisonous but can cause life-threatening allergic reactions in children with severe allergies to them (see Chapter 4 on anaphylactic shock).

When You See

- Complaints of pain, burning, or itching at sting site
- Redness, swelling
- Stinger possibly still in skin

Do This First

1. Remove the stinger from the skin by scraping it away gently with a rigid piece of plastic like a credit card. Call 9-1-1 if the child is known to be allergic to stings (see Chapter 4).
2. Wash the area with soap and water.
3. Put ice or a cold pack on the sting site.

4. Watch the child for 30 minutes for any signs or symptoms of allergic reaction (difficulty breathing, swelling in other areas, anxiety, nausea or vomiting); call 9-1-1 and treat for shock.

Additional Care

- Follow your childcare center's policy for using an over-the-counter oral antihistamine to help reduce discomfort or calamine to reduce itching. Parental permission is required.

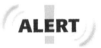

ALERT

Insect Sting in Mouth

Have the child suck on ice to reduce swelling. Call 9-1-1 if breathing becomes difficult.

Scorpion Stings

Scorpion stings are treated similarly to spider bites. Of the different types of scorpions in the American Southwest, some are more poisonous than others and could be dangerous, especially for young children. Antivenin may be available in some areas (**Figure 9-7**).

When You See

- The scorpion sting with its tail
- Complaints of severe burning pain at sting site, later numbness, tingling
- Nausea, vomiting
- Difficulty swallowing
- Possible convulsions, coma

Do This First

1. Call 9-1-1 if the child has trouble breathing.
2. Monitor the child's breathing and give BLS as needed.

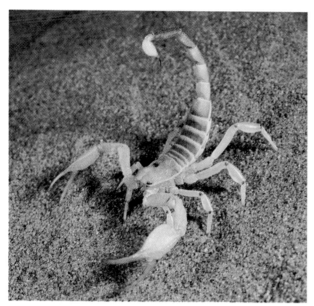

Figure 9-7 Scorpion.

3. Carefully wash the sting area.
4. Put ice or a cold pack on the area.
5. Seek urgent medical attention.

Additional Care

• Keep the child still.

Marine Bites and Stings

Biting marine animals include sharks, barracudas, and eels. Give this first aid for marine bites:

1. Stop the bleeding.
2. Care for shock.
3. Summon help from lifeguards.
4. Call 9-1-1.

Stinging marine life include jellyfish, Portuguese man-of-war, corals, and anemones. Give this first aid for marine animal stings:

1. Scrape off any tentacles on skin with a credit card or stick, or pick them off with tweezers or pliers.
2. Apply vinegar to the affected area.
3. Seek medical attention.

To care for stingray puncture wounds:

1. Relieve the pain by immersing the injured part in hot water for 30 minutes. Make sure the water is not so hot that it causes a burn.
2. Wash the wound with soap and water.
3. Seek medical attention.

10 Cold and Heat Emergencies

Cold or hot environments can cause medical problems for children if they are not protected from temperature extremes. Often cold- and heat-related injuries begin gradually, but if a child remains exposed to an extreme temperature, an emergency can develop. Untreated, it can lead to serious injury or death.

COLD INJURIES

Exposure to cold temperatures can cause either localized freezing of skin and other tissues (**frostnip** or **frostbite**) or lowering of the whole body's temperature below 95° Fahrenheit (**hypothermia**). Frostbite occurs when the temperature is 32° Fahrenheit or colder. Hypothermia can occur at much warmer temperatures if the body is unprotected, especially if the child is wet, exposed a long time, or unable to restore body heat because of a medical condition.

Frostbite

Frostbite is the freezing of skin or deeper tissues. It usually happens to exposed skin areas on the head or face, hands, or feet. Wind chill increases the risk of frostbite. Severe frostbite kills tissue and can result in gangrene and having to amputate the body part (**Figure 10-1**).

Frostnip is a less serious freezing of superficial skin areas, but it may progress to frostbite and become serious.

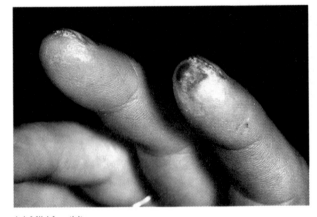

(a) Mild frostbite

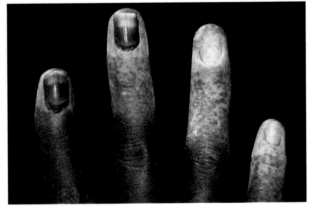

(b) Severe frostbite

Figure 10-1 Frostbite.

When You See

- Skin looks waxy and white, gray, yellow, or bluish.
- The area is numb or feels tingly or aching.
- With severe frostbite:
  - The area feels hard.
  - May become painless.
  - After warming, the area becomes swollen and may blister.

Do This First

1. Move the child to a warm environment. Gently hold the frostbitten area with your hands to warm it. (A child with frostbitten hands can warm them in his or her armpits.) Check the child also for hypothermia.
2. Remove any tight clothing or jewelry from the area.
3. Put dry gauze or fluffy cloth between frostbitten fingers or toes (**Figure 10-2**).
4. Obtain medical attention as soon as possible.
5. Additionally for severe frostbite:
   a. Only if medical care will be delayed and there is no risk of refreezing, warm the frostbitten area in lukewarm, not hot, water for at least 20 minutes or up to 45 minutes (**Figure 10-3**).
   b. Protect the area from being touched or rubbed by clothing or objects.
   c. Elevate the area if possible to reduce swelling.

Additional Care

- Follow your childcare center's policy for giving acetaminophen or ibuprofen for pain (parental permission required).
- Give the child a warm liquid to drink.
- Prevent the area from refreezing.

ALERT

Frostbite

Do not rub frostbitten skin because this can damage the skin.
Do not rewarm frostbitten skin if it may be frozen again, which could worsen the injury.
Do not use a fire, heat lamp, hot water bottle, or heating pad to warm the area.
After rewarming, be careful not to break blisters.

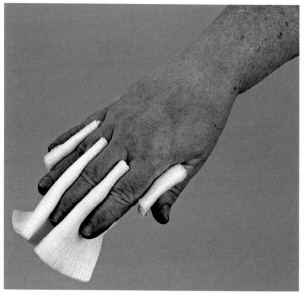

Figure 10-2 Protect between frostbitten fingers or toes.

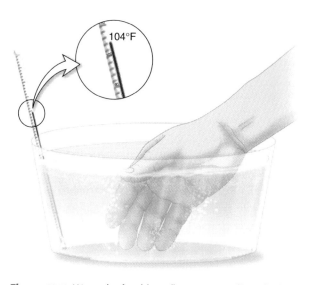

Figure 10-3 Warm the frostbitten fingers or toes if medical care will be delayed.

Hypothermia

When a child's body cannot make heat as fast as it loses it in a cold environment, the child develops hypothermia. In hypothermia, the body temperature drops below 95° Fahrenheit. Hypothermia can occur whenever and wherever the child feels cold, including indoors in poorly heated areas. It may occur gradually or quickly, especially with a wind chill or if the child is wet.

FACTS ABOUT HYPOTHERMIA

- Hypothermia occurs more easily in someone who is ill.
- A child immersed in cold water loses body heat 30 times faster than in cool air.
- A child in cold water is more likely to die from hypothermia than to drown.
- Children in cardiac arrest after immersion in cold water have been resuscitated after a long time underwater—don't give up!

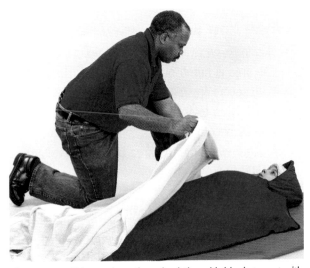

Figure 10-4 Warm a hypothermia victim with blankets, not with hot water.

When You See

- Shivering may be uncontrollable (but stops in severe hypothermia)
- Child seems apathetic, confused, or irrational; may be belligerent
- Lethargy, clumsy movements, drowsiness
- Pale, cool skin—even under clothing
- Slow breathing
- Changing levels of responsiveness

Do This First

1. With an unresponsive child, check for breathing and provide BLS as needed. Call 9-1-1 for any child with hypothermia.
2. Quickly get the child out of the cold and remove any wet clothing. Handle the child gently.
3. Have the child lie down, and cover him or her with blankets or warm clothing (Figure 10-4).

Additional Care

- Stay with the child until help arrives.

ALERT

Hypothermia

Do not immerse a child with hypothermia in hot water or use direct heat (hot water bottle, heat lamp, heating pad), because rapid warming can cause heart problems.

HEAT EMERGENCIES

Heat illnesses can result when children become overheated in a hot environment:

- *Heat cramps* are the least serious and usually first to occur.
- *Heat exhaustion* develops when the body becomes dehydrated in a hot environment.
- *Heatstroke,* with a seriously high body temperature, may develop from heat exhaustion. It is a medical emergency and, if untreated, usually causes death.

Heat Cramps

Activity in a hot environment may cause painful cramps in muscles, often in the lower legs or stomach muscles. Heat cramps may occur along with heat exhaustion and heatstroke.

When You See

- Signs of muscle pain, cramping, spasms
- Heavy sweating

Do This First

1. Have the child stop the activity and sit quietly in a cool place.
2. Give a sports drink or water.

Additional Care

- For abdominal cramps, continue resting in a comfortable position.
- For leg cramps, have the child stretch the muscle by extending the leg and flexing the ankle. Apply pressure to the cramped area.

Heat Exhaustion

Activity in a hot environment usually causes heavy sweating, which may lead to dehydration and depletion of salt and electrolytes in the body if the child does not get enough fluids. This situation could occur, for example, with a prolonged sports activity. Unrelieved, heat exhaustion may develop into heatstroke, a true medical emergency.

When You See

- Heavy sweating
- Thirst
- Fatigue
- Heat cramps

Later signs and symptoms:

- Headache, dizziness
- Nausea, vomiting

Do This First

1. Move the child out of the heat to rest in a cool place. Loosen or remove unnecessary clothing.

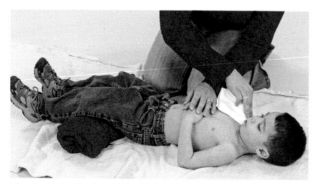

Figure 10-5 Cool a child with heat exhaustion.

2. Give a sports drink or water to drink.
3. Raise the legs 8 to 12 inches.
4. Cool the child by putting wet cloths on the forehead and body or sponging the skin with cool water (**Figure 10-5**).

Additional Care

- Seek medical care if the child's condition worsens or does not improve within 30 minutes.

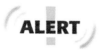

Heat Exhaustion

Do not give a child with heat exhaustion or heatstroke salt tablets. Use a sports drink instead (if the child is awake and alert). Do not give liquids containing caffeine. If the child is lethargic, nauseous, or vomiting, do not give any liquids.

Heatstroke

Heatstroke is a life-threatening emergency that is more common during hot summer periods. It may develop slowly over several days or more rapidly in someone engaged in strenuous activity in the heat. A child may be dehydrated and not sweating when heatstroke gradually develops, or may be sweating heavily from exertion. Heatstroke causes a body temperature of 104° Fahrenheit or higher and is different from heat exhaustion in these ways:

- In heatstroke the child's skin is flushed and feels very hot to the touch; in heat exhaustion the skin may be pale and clammy.
- In heatstroke the child becomes very confused and irrational and may become unresponsive or have convulsions; in heat exhaustion the child is dizzy or disoriented.

When You See

- Skin flushed and very hot to the touch, sweating may have stopped
- Fast breathing
- Headache, dizziness, confusion
- Irrational behavior
- Possible convulsions or unresponsiveness

Do This First

1. Call 9-1-1.
2. Move the child to a cool place and monitor his or her breathing.
3. Remove outer clothing.
4. Cool the child quickly with any means at hand:
   - Wrap the child in a wet sheet and keep it wet.
   - Sponge the child with cold water.
   - Spray the skin with water and then fan the area.
   - Put ice bags or cold packs beside the neck, armpits, and groin (**Figure 10-6**).

Additional Care

- Stay with the child and be prepared to give BLS if needed.

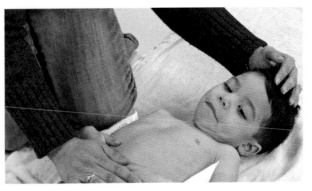

Figure 10-6 Cool a child with heatstroke.

- Put an unresponsive child who is breathing in the recovery position.
- Protect a child having convulsions from injury (see Chapter 8).

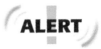

Heatstroke

A child with heatstroke should not take pain relievers or salt tablets.

Chapter

11 Common Minor Childhood Problems and Injuries

The childhood problems and injuries described in this chapter are seldom emergencies. Yet these are common problems that cause pain, discomfort, or other problems for children, and caregivers should know the first aid steps to take.

OBJECT IN EAR

Small children often put things in their ears, or an insect may crawl in while the child is sleeping. A child may be fussing with the ear or tell you there is something in it.

When You See

- Child is bothered by ear
- Child feels something moving in ear

Do This First

1. Look in the ear to see the object, but do not try to remove it. Only a healthcare provider should remove an object from the ear.
2. If you see or know an insect is in the ear, gently pour lukewarm water into the ear to try to float it out. If it does not come out, the child should see a healthcare provider.

Additional Care

- Reassure the child.

Action for parents:

- Take the child to a healthcare provider for removal of an object or insect that does not come out.

ALERT

Object in Ear

Never insert tweezers or anything else in a child's ear in an attempt to remove an object or insect, because of the risk of injury or pushing it farther in. See a healthcare provider.

OBJECT IN NOSE

A young child may have an object in the nose for some time before telling caregivers.

When You See

- Noisy or difficult breathing through nose
- Nasal discharge on one side
- Child may pick at nose with fingers
- Possible swelling of nose

Do This First

1. Look in the nose to see object, but do not try to remove it. Only a healthcare provider should remove an object from the nose, because of the risk of pushing it in farther.
2. Tell child to breathe through the mouth.

Additional Care

- Calm and reassure the child.

Action for parents:

- Take child to a healthcare provider for removal of the object.

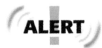

Object in Nose

Except with an older child skilled at blowing his or her nose, do not have the child try to expel an object from the nose by blowing it out. A young child may instead suck it in deeper.

SWALLOWED OBJECT

If the swallowed object is small and smooth, like a coin or button, it will usually pass through the child's system easily and safely. Any object that can dissolve may be poisonous, however (see Chapter 9). Be sure the object was swallowed and is not lodged in the windpipe, producing the signs of choking (see Chapter 2).

When You See

- You see or the child tells you he or she swallowed something

Do This First

1. Talk to the child to confirm what was swallowed.
2. With small, smooth, nonpoisonous objects, no action may be needed.
3. With objects that are larger or pointed or have rough edges, the child should see a healthcare provider. Do not give the child anything to eat or drink.

Additional Care

Actions for parents:

- Take the child to a healthcare provider for a large or sharp object.
- Call a healthcare provider if there is any question about the safety of the swallowed object.
- Observe the child for 3 to 4 days, and call the healthcare provider for any abdominal pain.

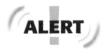

Swallowed Object

Do not try to induce vomiting or give a laxative to a child who swallows an object. Call a healthcare provider for advice if unsure about the safety of the swallowed object.

BUMP ON THE HEAD

Children often fall or run into things and bump their heads. With a more severe impact there may be bleeding or a more serious head injury (see Chapters 3 and 6). This section describes care for a minor bump not involving bleeding. The pain of such a bump usually does not last long.

When You See

- Child crying, holding head
- Swollen bump, often a large "goose egg"

Do This First

1. Calm and reassure the child.
2. Hold a covered ice or cold pack on the bump to minimize swelling and pain.
3. Monitor the child for any signs of a more serious injury. Call 9-1-1 immediately if the child becomes unresponsive or unusually lethargic, has enlarged pupils, vomits repeatedly, becomes very pale, or sweats heavily.

Additional Care

Action for parents:

- Continue to watch the child for development of any additional symptoms, and call a healthcare provider immediately if so.

SPLINTERS

Wooden splinters in a child are usually only a minor problem (**Figure 11-1**).

When You See

- A splinter in the child's skin

Do This First

1. Wash the area with soap and water.

2. Sterilize a pair of tweezers with alcohol or disinfectant and dry them. Grasp the splinter close to the skin and pull it out at the same angle.
3. Squeeze the skin around the area to promote bleeding to flush out the wound.
4. Wash the area again and apply a local antiseptic, if allowed. Cover the wound with an adhesive bandage.

Additional Care

- If the splinter is too deep to remove, apply antiseptic and bandage and wait for the splinter to work itself out in a day or two.

Action for parents:

- Talk to a healthcare provider if a part of the splinter remains beneath the skin.

ALERT

Splinter

Do not use a needle or knife to try to dig out a splinter beneath the skin.

TONGUE BITE

When a child bites his or her tongue, there may be significant bleeding at first. The situation usually looks scarier than it is.

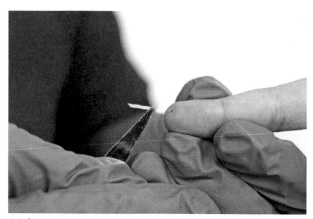

(a) Grasp a splinter close to the skin.

Figure 11-1 Removing a splinter.

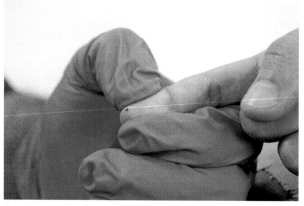

(b) Squeeze the skin around the area to promote bleeding.

When You See

- Child's tongue bleeding

Do This First

1. Have child spit out the blood rather than swallow it.
2. Rinse mouth with cold water.
3. Wearing gloves, press a piece of clean gauze on the wound to control the bleeding.

Additional Care

- A cold pack on the lips or tongue may help reduce pain and swelling.
- Do not let child eat or drink anything for a while.

Action for parents:

- Call a healthcare provider if the bleeding does not stop soon or the wound seems deep.

FINGERNAIL INJURY

When a child smashes a finger, the fingernail may be partly or completely torn away, or there may be bleeding beneath the nail. The injury usually looks worse than it is, however, and except in very severe injuries the nail will grow back over four to sixteen weeks.

When You See

- Bleeding around and under a fingernail or toenail
- The nail torn partly or completely away

Do This First

1. Check that the child can move the finger or joints; a possible fracture should be seen by a healthcare provider.
2. Gently wash or rinse the nail area to clean it.
3. Leave the damaged nail in place.
4. Use an ice or cold pack to reduce swelling and pain.

Additional Care

- Follow your center's policy for giving children's acetaminophen or ibuprofen for pain if needed (parental permission required).

Actions for parents:

- Call a healthcare provider if the pressure of blood trapped under the nail causes pain.
- Keep the fingernail bandaged as long as it is painful or if a ragged edge may catch and tear the remaining nail.

LOSING A BABY TOOTH

New parents and caregivers sometimes worry about children losing their baby teeth and swallowing or choking on them. In reality this very rarely happens, although it may be a concern if a child's tooth is knocked out by a blow. In this case, be sure the tooth is not caught in the child's throat; if so, give first aid for choking (see Chapter 2).

If a baby tooth that was not loose is knocked out, the child's dentist should be called, because in some cases the dentist may want to reimplant the tooth. If so, control bleeding in the child and care for the tooth (see Chapter 3).

When You See

- A child loses a baby tooth that was loose

Do This First

1. Have child spit out the blood rather than swallow it.
2. Rinse mouth with cold water.
3. Wearing gloves, put a rolled or folded piece of clean gauze over the tooth socket and apply gentle pressure to control bleeding.

Additional Care

- Do not let child eat or drink anything for a while.
- Save the tooth for the child's parents.

BLISTERS

Blisters usually occur because of friction on the skin, such as if a child's shoe rubs the back of the ankle or heel. They can be painful and may become infected after breaking. Burns may cause a different kind of blister (see Chapter 5).

When You See

- A raised, fluid-filled blister, often surrounded by red skin

Do This First

1. Wash the blister and surrounding area with soap and water. Rinse and gently pat dry.
2. Cover the blister with an adhesive bandage big enough that the gauze pad covers the whole blister. Bandages with an adhesive strip on all four sides are best because they keep the area cleaner if the blister breaks.

Additional Care

- Prevent continued friction in the area.

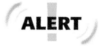

Blister
Never deliberately break a blister.
This could lead to infection.

Chapter

12 Child Abuse and Neglect

Child abuse and neglect are major problems in our society. Over 2,000 children a day are discovered to be victims of child abuse or neglect. Each week, child protective service agencies throughout the United States receive more than 50,000 reports of suspected child abuse or neglect. Every year over 800,000 children are found to have been victims of abuse or neglect. About two-thirds of these children are experiencing neglect, meaning a caretaker failed to provide for their basic needs. Almost 20% are found to have been physically abused, and about 10% sexually abused. About 8% are victims of emotional abuse, which includes criticizing, rejecting, or refusing to nurture a child. An average of three children die every day as a result of child abuse or neglect.

Childcare workers, teachers, and parents all need to understand the nature of this problem and what they can do for children being abused.

Much of the information in this chapter comes from the National Clearinghouse on Child Abuse and Neglect Information, of the U.S. Department of Health and Human Services Administration for Children and Families. Additional information is available at this agency's website: http://nccanch.acf.hhs.gov.

WHY ABUSE OCCURS

All the causes of child abuse and neglect are not fully understood, but several risk factors have been identified. When there are multiple risk factors present, the risk is greater. These risk factors include:

- Lack of preparation or knowledge for parenting

- Financial or other environmental stressors
- Difficulty in relationships
- Depression or other mental health problems

Parents may lack an understanding of their children's developmental stages and hold unreasonable expectations for their abilities. They also may be unaware of alternatives to corporal punishment or how to discipline their children most effectively at each age. Parents also may lack knowledge of the health, hygiene, and nutritional needs of their children. These circumstances, combined with the challenges of raising children, can result in otherwise well-intentioned parents causing their children harm or neglecting their needs.

Abuse may also result from uncontrolled emotional states. A particular problem, for example, is **shaken baby syndrome,** in which a parent or caregiver, including babysitters and childcare workers, becomes frustrated with a crying infant and shakes the infant. Such shaking causes the infant's head to flop around and may cause severe brain injury, spinal injury, or death. Everyone who cares for infants needs to understand this problem and to learn to control their emotions when frustrated by the crying of a child.

WHO IS ABUSED

Any child may be abused. Boys and girls are almost equally likely to experience neglect and physical abuse. Girls are four times more likely to experience sexual abuse. Children of all races and ethnicities and all socioeconomic levels experience abuse.

Children of all ages experience abuse and neglect, but younger children are most vulnerable. Infants under 1 year old account for nearly one-half of deaths resulting from child abuse and neglect, and about 85% of children who die are younger than 6 years of age.

Mothers acting alone are responsible for almost half the cases of neglect and about one-third of the cases of physical abuse. Fathers acting alone are responsible for about one-fourth of cases of sexual abuse, and unrelated perpetrators about one-third of cases of sexual abuse. In about 80% of cases of sexual abuse, the perpetrator is known by the child. Often sexual abuse occurs in a pattern rather than a single incident.

TYPES OF ABUSE AND NEGLECT

The **Federal Child Abuse Prevention and Treatment Act,** amended by the Keeping Children and Families Safe Act of 2003, defines child abuse and neglect as, at minimum:

- Any recent act or failure to act on the part of a parent or caretaker which results in death, serious physical or emotional harm, sexual abuse or exploitation; or
- An act or failure to act which presents an imminent risk of serious harm.

Each state, however, has its own laws and exact definitions of child abuse and neglect, which are typically based on the national standard. Most states recognize four major types of maltreatment: neglect, physical abuse, sexual abuse, and emotional abuse. Although any of these types may occur separately, they are more often combined. For example, a physically abused child is often emotionally abused as well, and a sexually abused child also may be neglected.

Neglect

Neglect is failure to provide for a child's basic needs, including these forms of neglect:

- *Physical neglect.* Failure to provide necessary food or shelter, or a lack of appropriate supervision.
- *Medical neglect.* Failure to provide necessary medical or mental health treatment.
- *Educational neglect.* Failure to educate a child or attend to special education needs.
- *Emotional neglect.* Inattention to a child's emotional needs, failure to provide psychological care, or permitting the child to use alcohol or other drugs.

These situations do not always mean a child is willfully neglected, however. Sometimes cultural values, community standards, and poverty may be contributing factors. The family may need information or assistance. When a family fails to use information and resources, and the child's health or safety is at risk, then child welfare intervention may be required.

Physical Abuse

Physical abuse is physical injury (ranging from minor bruises to severe fractures or death) as a result of punching, beating, kicking, biting, shaking, throwing, stabbing, choking, hitting (with a hand, stick, strap, or other object), burning, or otherwise harming a child. These injuries are considered abuse regardless of whether the caretaker intended to hurt the child.

Sexual Abuse

Sexual abuse includes any kind of sexual activity by a parent or caretaker, such as fondling a child's genitals, penetration, incest, rape, sodomy, indecent exposure, or exploitation through prostitution or the production of pornographic materials.

Emotional Abuse

Emotional abuse is a pattern of behavior that impairs a child's emotional development or sense of self-worth. This may include constant criticism, threats, or rejection, as well as withholding love, support, or guidance. Emotional abuse is often difficult to prove, and government agencies often cannot intervene without evidence of harm to the child. Emotional abuse is almost always present when other types of abuse occur.

RESULTS OF ABUSE AND NEGLECT

Abuse and neglect have short- and long-term consequences that may include brain damage, developmental delays, learning disorders, problems forming relationships, aggressive behavior, and depression. Survivors of child abuse and neglect may also be at greater risk for problems later in life, such as low academic achievement, drug use, teen pregnancy, and criminal behavior.

SIGNS OF ABUSE AND NEGLECT

The first step in helping abused or neglected children is learning to recognize the signs of abuse and neglect. A single sign does not prove child abuse is occurring, but when signs appear repeatedly or in combination, you should consider the possibility of child abuse.

General Signs of Abuse

Behavioral signs may signal abuse or neglect long before any physical changes occur in a child. The following behaviors may suggest the possibility of child abuse or neglect:

The child:
- Has sudden changes in behavior or school performance
- Has not received help for physical or medical problems brought to the parents' attention
- Has learning problems or difficulty concentrating unrelated to specific physical or psychological causes
- Is always watchful, as though preparing for something bad to happen
- Lacks adult supervision
- Is overly compliant, passive, or withdrawn
- Comes to school or other activities early, stays late, and does not want to go home

The parent:
- Shows little concern for the child
- Denies the existence of—or blames the child for—the child's problems in school or at home
- Asks teachers or other caretakers to use harsh physical discipline if the child misbehaves
- Sees the child as entirely bad, worthless, or burdensome
- Demands a level of physical or academic performance the child cannot achieve
- Looks primarily to the child for care, attention, and satisfaction of emotional needs

The parent and child:
- Rarely touch or look at each other
- Consider their relationship entirely negative
- Say they do not like each other

Signs of Neglect

The child:
- Is frequently absent from school
- Begs or steals food or money
- Lacks needed medical or dental care, immunizations, or glasses
- Is consistently dirty and has severe body odor
- Lacks sufficient clothing for the weather

- Abuses alcohol or other drugs
- Says there is no one at home to provide care

The parent or other adult caregiver:
- Appears indifferent to the child
- Seems apathetic or depressed
- Behaves irrationally or in a bizarre manner
- Is abusing alcohol or other drugs

See the box below for specific signs of the different types of abuse.

SIGNS OF ABUSE

Signs of Physical Abuse
The child:
- Has unexplained scalding or burns, rope burns, lacerations, bites, bruises, broken bones, or black eyes
- Has fading bruises or other marks after an absence from school or childcare
- Seems frightened of parents and protests or cries when it is time to go home
- Shrinks at the approach of adults
- Reports being injured by a parent or another adult caregiver
- Appears withdrawn or depressed and cries often—or is aggressive and disruptive
- Seems tired often and complains of frequent nightmares

The parent or other adult caregiver:
- Offers conflicting, unconvincing, or no explanation for the child's injury
- Describes the child with words such as "evil" or other negative terms
- Uses harsh physical discipline with the child
- Is known to have a history of abuse as a child

Signs of Sexual Abuse
The child:
- Has difficulty walking or sitting
- Suddenly refuses to change clothing when necessary or to participate in physical activities

- Reports nightmares or bedwetting
- Experiences a sudden change in appetite
- Demonstrates bizarre, sophisticated, or unusual sexual knowledge or behavior
- Becomes pregnant or contracts a venereal disease, particularly if under age 14
- Runs away from home
- Reports sexual abuse by a parent or other adult caregiver
- Seems afraid of a particular person or being alone with that person

The parent or other adult caregiver:
- Is unduly protective of the child or severely limits the child's contact with other children, especially of the opposite sex
- Is secretive and isolated
- Is jealous or controlling with family members

Signs of Emotional Abuse
The child:
- Is extreme in behavior, such as overly compliant or demanding, extremely passive or aggressive
- Acts either inappropriately like an adult (such as parenting other children) or inappropriately like an infant (such as frequently rocking or head-banging)
- Has delayed physical or emotional development
- Has attempted suicide
- Demonstrates a lack of attachment to the parent

The parent or other adult caregiver:
- Constantly blames, belittles, or berates the child
- Seems unconcerned about the child and refuses to consider offers of help for the child's problems
- Overtly rejects the child

Helping an Abused Child

Parents or other caregivers who abuse or neglect a child need help. Programs are available in most communities to provide professional help.

Childcare workers, teachers, and other caregivers should not, however, try to talk to suspected abusers in an effort to get them to seek help. Almost always the abuser will deny the problem, and the situation may become worse than if you had said nothing. Instead, the single most important thing you can do, if you suspect a child is being abused or neglected, is report it to the proper authorities. Your report will help protect the child and get help for the family.

Reporting Abuse

If you care for children as part of your job, you may be legally required to report suspected cases of child abuse or neglect. State laws vary in the specifics of who must make a report and to what agency. If this is required in your job, follow your employer's policy. For example, you may be required to speak to your supervisor about your suspicion before making a report.

The law provides ways for private citizens to report suspected abuse or neglect as well, and it is important for the child's welfare that you do this even if not required to do so by your employer. Contact your local child protective services agency or police department. For more information about where and how to file a report, call the Childhelp USA® National Child Abuse Hotline (1-800-4-A-CHILD).

When you call to report child abuse, you will be asked for specific information, which may include:

- The child's name
- The suspected perpetrator's name (if known)
- A description of what you have seen or heard
- The names of any other people having knowledge of the abuse
- Your name and phone number

Your name will not be given to the family of the child you suspect is being abused or neglected. If you are making the report as a private citizen, you may request to make the report anonymously, but your report may be considered more credible and can be more helpful to the child protective services agency if you give your name.

Remember: Your suspicion of child abuse or neglect is enough to make a report. You do not have to provide proof. Almost every state has a law to protect people who make good-faith reports of child abuse from prosecution or liability.

What Happens When a Report Is Made

When a report is made it will first be screened by the agency. If the agency determines there is enough credible information to indicate that maltreatment may have occurred or is at risk of occurring, an investigation will be conducted. Depending on the potential severity of the situation, investigators may respond within hours or days. They may speak with the child, the parents, and other people in contact with the child, such as healthcare providers, teachers, or childcare providers.

If the investigator feels the child is at risk of harm, the family may be referred to any of various programs to reduce the risk of future maltreatment. These may include mental health care, medical care, parenting skills classes, employment assistance, and support services such as financial or housing assistance. In rare cases where the child's safety cannot be ensured, the child may be removed from the home.

The best way to prevent child abuse and neglect is to support families and provide parents with the skills and resources they need. Prevention efforts build on family strengths. Through activities such as parent education, home visitation, and parent support groups, many families are able to find the support they need to stay together and care for their children in their homes and communities. Prevention efforts help parents develop their parenting skills, understand the benefits of nonviolent discipline techniques, and understand and meet their child's emotional, physical, and developmental needs.

First Aid for an Apparently Abused Child

If you suspect a child in your care is being abused or neglected, do not confront the parents or ask the child direct questions about abuse. If the child needs first aid for an illness or injury, provide it as you would for any child, following the standard guidelines for providing care. Follow your facility's guidelines for documenting the care and any additional actions. If the child tells you an injury was caused by a parent or other adult, include this information when making your report.

13 Common Childhood Illnesses

Children frequently experience common illnesses because their immune systems are not yet fully developed and because infections spread among children quickly in indoor settings such as schools and childcare centers. Fortunately, most childhood illnesses are not serious, although a few can become medical emergencies. The spread of viral and bacterial illness can be minimized with good ventilation and preventive practices such as frequent handwashing, early recognition and treatment of illness, and keeping a sick child home from school or childcare. Whenever a child is suspected of having an infectious disease, be sure to follow universal precautions to prevent transmission of the disease to others (see Chapter 1).

COLDS

Common colds generally last 5 to 10 days. Colds are transmitted from one person to another, not caught by getting cold or wet. Colds are most contagious during the first few days. Cold medicines do not cure or shorten colds but may offer some relief from symptoms. Causes include respiratory viruses.

When You See

- Sore throat, coughing
- Sneezing, stuffy or running nose
- Red, watery eyes
- Headache, body aches, and pains
- Fever

Do This First

1. Treat symptoms with children's cough medicine and decongestants if needed (not aspirin).

Parental permission required.
2. Use a cool-mist humidifier or vaporizer to minimize congestion.
3. Give plenty of fluids.
4. Do not let child share toys or eating utensils.

Additional Care

- Teach child to blow nose, use tissues when sneezing, and cover mouth when coughing.
- Teach child to wash hands often.

Actions for parents:

- Call a healthcare provider if fever becomes high or prolonged, if ears hurt, if the child is breathing rapidly, or if sore throat becomes severe.
- The child may attend school or childcare when a fever is under control and the child does not have nausea or diarrhea.

Sore Throat

Sore throat may be a symptom of a cold or something as simple as sleeping with the mouth open, or a more serious condition such as strep throat. Most sore throats are caused by viruses and are contagious.

Causes include:

- Viruses
- Strep bacteria
- Sleeping with mouth open

When You See

- Throat pain
- Swelling and redness of throat tissue
- Feeling tired
- Possible fever
- Possible difficulty swallowing or breathing

Do This First

1. Have child drink warm liquids and gargle frequently with warm salt water.
2. Use a cool-mist vaporizer to minimize pain.
3. Do not let child share toys or eating utensils.
4. See a healthcare provider for high or prolonged fever or for difficulty swallowing or breathing because of severe throat pain, or if the child breaks out in a skin rash.

Additional Care

- Follow your center's policy for giving children's acetaminophen or ibuprofen for pain (parental permission required).

Actions for parents:
- See a healthcare provider for fever, skin rash, or severe throat pain (antibiotics may be needed).
- A child with strep throat may return to school or childcare after 24 hours of antibiotic therapy if fever is gone.

Whooping Cough

Coughing is frequently a sign of a cold (see Colds section earlier) or other respiratory infection but may also occur with **whooping cough** (pertussis). Care for a child with whooping cough is described in this section.

Whooping cough is contagious. Young children are usually given a pertussis vaccine, but immunity may not last indefinitely.

Causes include:

- Bacterial infection

When You See

- In early stage: sneezing, nasal congestion, coughing
- Later stage (may last several weeks): uncontrollable bouts of coughing with whooping sound on inhalation

Do This First

1. Do not let child share toys or eating utensils.
2. A child suspected of having whooping cough should see a healthcare provider as soon as possible.

Additional Care

- Healthcare providers must report positive whooping cough cases.
- Parents of other children in contact with sick child should be notified.

Actions for parents:
- Take child to see a healthcare provider (antibiotic will be given).
- The healthcare provider will advise when child can return to school or childcare.

Ear Infection

Middle-ear infections are the most common cause of ear pain in infants and young children, diminishing as the child grows older. Congestion in the eustachian tube, such as occurs with a cold, allows bacteria to grow. The infection puts pressure on the ear drum, causing pain. Ear infections are not contagious.

Causes include:

- Bacterial or viral infection

When You See

- Ear pain, pulling at or rubbing ear
- Irritability
- Possible fever
- Possible drainage from ear

Do This First

1. Follow your center's policy for giving children's acetaminophen or ibuprofen for pain (parental permission required).
2. Keep child upright to reduce pain.

Additional Care

- A covered hot water bottle or heating pad may help relieve pain.

Actions for parents:

- Take child to see a healthcare provider (antibiotic will be given).
- Child can return to school or childcare when feeling well enough and fever has subsided.

CHICKEN POX

Chicken pox is a common contagious disease that spreads easily among children. Chicken pox can cause considerable discomfort but seldom is a serious condition. A vaccine is available and is recommended for school-age children who have not had chicken pox. Having chicken pox confers immunity (**Figure 13-1**).

Causes include:

- Viral infection

When You See

- A skin rash of itchy red spots, mostly on trunk and face
- Rash bumps break open, weep, then scab over
- Fever

Do This First

1. Keep child from scratching open the rash bumps.
2. Use calamine lotion or colloidal oatmeal for itching.
3. Keep child away from nonimmunized other children.

Additional Care

- Follow your center's policy for giving children's acetaminophen or ibuprofen for fever if needed (parental permission required).

Actions for parents:

- See a healthcare provider for high or persistent fever, rapid breathing, or other severe symptoms.
- The child may return to school or childcare when all of the rash has dried and crusted.

CONJUNCTIVITIS (PINKEYE)

Conjunctivitis, commonly called pinkeye, is an infection of the membranes inside the eyelids. This condition is contagious but usually not serious (**Figure 13-2**).

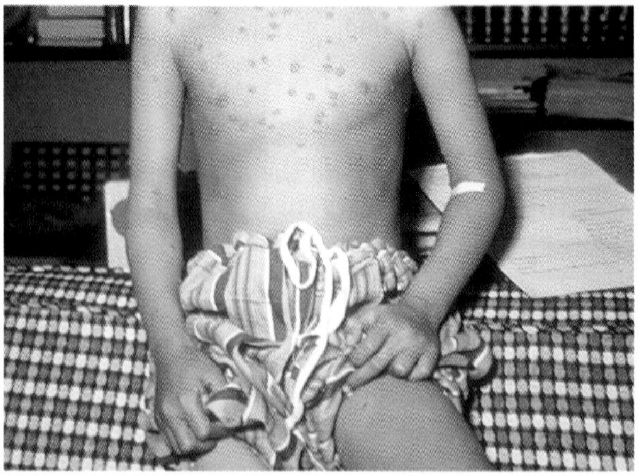

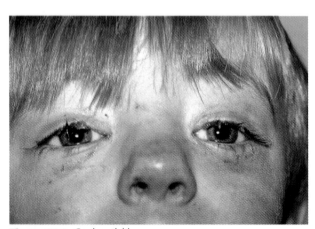

Figure 13-1 Chicken pox.

Figure 13-2 Conjunctivitis.

Causes include:

- Viral infection
- Bacterial infection
- Severe allergic condition

When You See

- One or both eyes look pink or red
- Yellow, green, or clear pus or drainage from eye(s)
- Eyelids may stick together after sleeping

Do This First

1. Keep child from rubbing eyes.
2. Child and others should wash hands frequently.
3. Do not let child share toys or eating utensils.
4. Carefully wash drainage from eyes with cotton ball or gauze soaked in warm water.

Additional Care

Actions for parents:

- See a healthcare provider since bacterial infection requires an antibiotic.
- The child can return to school or childcare when drainage from the eyes stops, often after 1 to 2 days on an antibiotic.

HEADACHE

Headaches are common in children. Headache may result from simple stress or fatigue, from various common illnesses such as a cold or the flu, or more rarely from a serious problem such as meningitis (see Chapter 8) or a head injury (see Chapter 6). Children may also have migraine headaches, which are recurring, severe, throbbing, or stabbing headaches that may involve nausea and vomiting.

With a sudden, severe, unexplained headache, always look for a more serious cause. The following care is for nonemergency minor headaches.

Causes include:

- A cold or other infection
- Stress, fatigue
- Eye strain

When You See

- Child complains his or her head hurts
- Child may be holding head

Do This First

1. Have child rest quietly in darkened room.
2. Follow your center's policy for giving children's acetaminophen or ibuprofen (parental permission required).
3. Be alert for other symptoms.

Additional Care

Actions for parents:

- See a healthcare provider for recurring or severe headaches or for headache with stiff neck, marked irritability or lethargy, visual problems, a purple spotted rash, or repeated vomiting.
- Child may attend school or childcare.

DIARRHEA

Diarrhea in children is common and may result from a variety of different infections and conditions. Most often a viral infection of the stomach or intestines is the cause. Diarrhea can also result from other causes, including bacteria that are very contagious. Caregivers should wear gloves when changing diapers and wash hands frequently. When caused by infection, diarrhea may last several days to a week.

Causes include:

- Viral or bacterial infection
- Intestinal parasites
- Dietary changes
- Antibiotics

When You See

- Frequent loose, watery, or mushy stools
- Child may also vomit

Do This First

1. Keep the child well hydrated:
   a. Give an infant an electrolyte solution (such as Pedialyte) between breast feedings; do not give infant formula for one or two feedings.
   b. Give a child an electrolyte solution (such as Pedialyte) or a half-and-half mixture of a sports drink and water.
   c. If drinking fluids seems to increase vomiting, give fluid in small amounts frequently; have the child suck on ice chips.
2. With an infant, change the diaper immediately and wash the anal area well. A commercial product may minimize skin irritation.
3. Feed the child foods that minimize diarrhea, such as dry toast, bananas, crackers, applesauce (but not apple juice), rice, dry cereals, and other low-fat foods. Avoid milk, butter and margarine, cheese, and ice cream.

Additional Care

- Make sure the child uses good hygiene habits and washes hands well after using the bathroom.

Actions for parents:

Call a healthcare provider and ask him or her when the child can return to school or childcare:

- If the diarrhea contains blood, pus, or mucus
- For an infant under 6 months old
- If the child seems dehydrated or very sick
- If the child cannot drink
- If the diarrhea lasts more than 3 days

CONSTIPATION

Constipation in children is usually temporary and not a sign of a serious condition. Constipation may occur, however, if another illness causes fever and vomiting that leads to dehydration.

Causes include:

- Changes in diet
- Not enough fiber in diet
- Dehydration or not drinking enough fluids

When You See

- Difficult bowel movements
- Hard, dry feces

Do This First

1. Have the child drink plenty of fluids.
2. Ensure that the child's diet includes fruits and vegetables and other fiber-rich foods.

Additional Care

- For a toddler in toilet training, encourage child not to avoid bowel movements.

Action for parents:

- See a healthcare provider if the child still has constipation after a week or has not had a bowel movement in 4 days.

ALERT

Constipation

Do not give a child a laxative unless instructed by the healthcare provider.

STOMACHACHE

Stomachaches are common in young children, and some children may complain frequently. Usually the stomachache results from something minor, but occasionally the child may have a serious medical condition. Always monitor the child for other symptoms that may suggest a more serious condition (see Chapter 8). Also see the next section in this chapter, on vomiting.

Causes include:

- Overeating
- Gas
- Stomach or intestinal infections
- Appendicitis and certain rare medical conditions

When You See

- Child complaining of stomach pain
- Child may be holding or rubbing stomach

Do This First

1. Have the child rest or lie down for 15 minutes.
2. Have the child hold a covered hot water bottle or heating pad on the stomach if this eases the pain.
3. Have a bowl or basin handy in case the child vomits.
4. Observe child for other symptoms.

Additional Care

- Do not give the child food (clear fluids are okay).

Actions for parents:

Call a healthcare provider if:

- The pain seems severe.
- The pain lasts longer than 2 hours, or comes and goes for more than 12 hours.
- Stomachaches are frequent.
- The child vomits blood or a black or green substance.
- There is blood in the stool.
- The child has a high fever or signs of appendicitis.

When You See

- Child seems nauseous or says stomach hurts

Do This First

1. Be prepared for vomiting with a bowl or basin. Hold the child over the basin.
2. After the child vomits, wash around the mouth.
3. Do not give food or fluid for up to an hour, then let child slowly sip water or suck on ice chips.

Additional Care

- Let child rest or lie down, but do not feed right away. When the child is ready to eat, give bland foods (same as for diarrhea).
- Wear gloves when giving care, and wash hands afterwards. Have child also wash hands.

Actions for parents:

Call a healthcare provider:

- For an infant under 6 months old
- If vomiting continues for 6 hours or more
- If the child has abdominal pain or fever
- If there is blood in the vomit
- If the child becomes dehydrated

VOMITING

Vomiting, like nausea or stomachache, is usually a symptom of a viral infection. Diarrhea may also occur (see earlier sections on stomachache and diarrhea). As with diarrhea, the most important care is to prevent dehydration. The infection may be contagious.

Note that infants often "spit up" after being fed, particularly if not burped. This is not the same as vomiting, and the infant usually quickly recovers. An infant's repeated vomiting, however, can quickly lead to dehydration and become a medical emergency; in this case the infant should be taken to the hospital.

Causes include:

- Stomach or intestinal viral infection
- Dietary changes

URINARY TRACT INFECTION

Urinary tract infections occur when bacteria from the skin, gastrointestinal tract, or environment get into the urinary tract. These infections can be painful and uncomfortable but rarely become serious. Urinary tract infections are more common in girls than in boys. Occasionally painful urination may occur with something other than a urinary tract infection, and a child needs to see a healthcare provider right away if there is also vomiting, back pain, fever, or shaking chills.

Causes include:

- Bacterial infection

When You See

- Pain, burning, or stinging on urination
- More frequent urination
- Possibly discolored urine

Do This First

1. Encourage the child to drink lots of fluids.
2. Ensure that the child sees a healthcare provider.

Additional Care

Prevent urinary tract infections by:

- Teaching girls to wipe from front to back after going to the bathroom
- Not using bubble baths or strong soaps
- Having child wear only cotton underwear

Actions for parents:

- Take the child to a healthcare provider (antibiotic treatment is needed).
- The child can attend school or childcare.

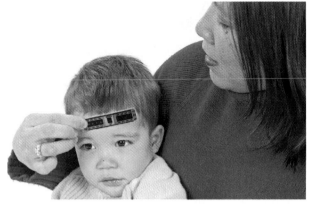

(a) Temperature strip

FEVER

Fever occurs often with viral or bacterial infections ranging from colds to ear infections and sore throats. Fever is a sign the body is fighting the infection. A rapidly rising fever in a child can cause a seizure (see Chapter 8) or in an infant can cause dehydration.

Although temperature strips may be used on the forehead for infants or very small children, they are not as accurate as thermometers either in the mouth (over age 4) or armpit (Figure 13-3). If possible, use a rectal thermometer for an infant (for 1 minute). Allow 3 minutes for oral measurement or 10 for the armpit. Digital thermometers usually need only 1 minute for a reading.

The normal oral temperature is 98.6 degrees Fahrenheit. The normal underarm temperature is 1 degree lower, the normal rectal temperature 1 degree higher.

Causes include:

- Viral or bacterial infection
- Heat exhaustion or heatstroke (see Chapter 10)
- Some medications or poisons (see Chapter 9)
- Extreme exertion

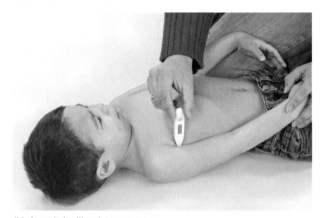

(b) Armpit (axillary) temperature

Figure 13-3 Checking for fever.

When You See

- A child's temperature more than 1 or 2 degrees above normal

Do This First

1. Since the child may have a contagious disease, have him or her rest away from other children.
2. Give the child lots of clear fluids.
3. For a fever over 101 degrees Fahrenheit, follow your center's policy for giving children's acetaminophen or ibuprofen if needed for the child's comfort (parental permission required).
4. For a fever over 103 degrees Fahrenheit, cool the child by sponging the skin with room-temperature water; avoid chilling.

Additional Care

- Observe the child for other symptoms and treat accordingly.

Actions for parents:

See a healthcare provider if:

- An infant under 3 months old has a fever above 100 degrees Fahrenheit.
- The fever lasts more than 24 hours in a child under 12 months old.
- An older child's fever is 104 degrees Fahrenheit or higher.
- Any fever lasts more than 5 days.
- The child has other serious symptoms such as a stiff neck, confusion, extreme irritability or lethargy, severe sore throat or headache, ear pain, repeated diarrhea or vomiting, or rapid breathing.
- The child can return to school or childcare 24 hours after the fever ends, or when approved by the healthcare provider.

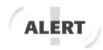

ALERT

Fever

Do not give a child aspirin because of the danger of Reye syndrome. Follow your center's policy for giving children's acetaminophen or ibuprofen if needed (parental permission required).

Diaper Rash

Diaper rash is a common, often painful skin irritation caused by exposure to wet diapers (**Figure 13-4**). It can be prevented by frequently changing a child's diaper and using good hygiene practices. The rash usually clears up in 2 to 3 days. Occasionally a more severe infection may occur, extending outside the diaper area or causing blisters.

Causes include:

- Wet diapers

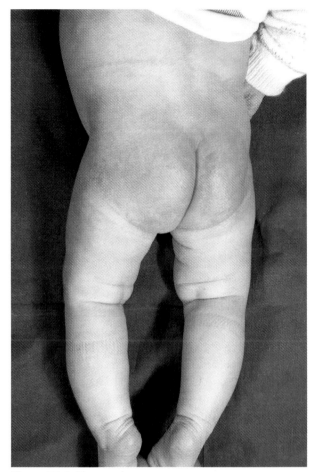

Figure 13-4 Diaper rash.

When You See

- A red rash in the diaper area
- Pain in the area

Do This First

1. Keep the skin dry by changing diapers often; do not use plastic pants. Leave diapers off as long as possible between changing.
2. Wash the area with mild soap and water. Soaking in water may help. Dry thoroughly before putting on a fresh diaper.
3. Rash may be prevented with zinc oxide, ointment, or petroleum jelly, but do not put ointment on an existing rash (may delay healing). Do not use baby powder or talc because of the risk of the infant inhaling it.

Additional Care

- Wear gloves when changing diapers, and wash hands afterward.
- Rinse cloth diapers with vinegar solution to remove irritating ammonia.

Actions for parents:

- Call a healthcare provider if blisters are present, the rash is outside the diaper area, or the rash continues longer than 3 days.
- The child can attend school or childcare.

COLD SORE

Cold sores are oozing blisters that can form anywhere on the body but are most common on the lips or inside the mouth. The infection is transmitted by contact, including through saliva, and cannot be cured. After the initial infection the virus stays inside the person, and cold sores reappear occasionally. An outbreak may be triggered by many factors, including cold or heat, stress, or fever. The sores form scabs and heal in 1 to 2 weeks (**Figure 13-5**).

Causes include:

- The herpes simplex virus

When You See

- Watery blisters on or near lips or in mouth
- Pain or itching

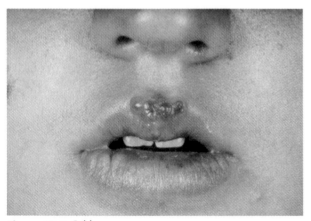

Figure 13-5 Cold sore.

Do This First

1. Keep child from picking at or scratching the sores.
2. Child and caregivers should wash hands frequently.
3. Relieve discomfort with lip balm.

Additional Care

Actions for parents:

- A young child who is likely to touch the sores and spread the virus to others should be kept home until the sores are scabbed over, unless they can be covered.
- An older child who understands the importance of not touching the sores can attend school or childcare.

TOOTHACHE

Toothache usually results from teething or cavities. A very young child may have tooth decay caused by having a bottle of milk or something sweet before naps or bedtime; this is sometimes called "bottlemouth." A child may sometimes not be able to identify the source of pain, however, and may have an earache, sore throat, or other condition. Watch for other symptoms that may suggest a medical rather than dental problem.

Causes include:

- Tooth decay, cavities
- New teeth coming through

When You See

- Tooth pain
- Possible low fever

Do This First

1. Inspect the mouth for any obvious problems. A swollen jaw and redness around the tooth may indicate an abscess that needs to be seen by a healthcare provider.

2. Follow your center's policy for giving children's acetaminophen or ibuprofen for pain (parental permission required). For teething pain, other commercial products may help.

3. Have child lie down with jaw against a covered hot water bottle or heating pad.

Additional Care

Actions for parents:

- Make a dental appointment for the child.
- See a healthcare provider if the child also has an earache or fever of 102 degrees Fahrenheit or higher.
- Without fever, the child can attend school or childcare.

Skin Rashes

Skin rashes and problems that cause rashes occur often in children. More than a dozen different common ailments can produce skin conditions loosely called a rash, making it often difficult to know for sure what is causing the child's skin problem. Fortunately, most skin problems are minor.

You cannot always, and sometimes not even usually, diagnose a rash based solely on its appearance, because there are so many different causes and the appearance may vary from child to child. The diagnosis often depends on other information, including:

- How the rash began
- Where it appears on the body
- How it spread
- Associated symptoms such as itching or fever
- Factors to which the child has been exposed

Treatment guidelines are based on the severity of the child's symptoms and the cause of the rash. Minor rashes that cause only minor discomfort may not require any treatment beyond observation. More serious rashes may be contagious or cause symptoms troubling enough to require treatment.

The following information is intended only as general information. Unless you are sure of the cause of a child's rash based on your experience, leave the diagnosis and treatment decisions to a healthcare provider.

Causes include:

- *Prickly heat* (heat rash). More common in very young children, little red bumps appear at sweat glands; treated by keeping child in cooler, less humid environment.
- *Diaper rash.* See earlier section in this chapter.
- *Hives.* An allergic reaction caused by certain foods, medications, even stress; can be emergency if breathing difficulty occurs (see Allergic Reactions in Chapter 4).
- *Poison ivy.* See Chapter 9.
- *Eczema.* A condition of dry, itching skin, often with family history, that may make young children scratch and cause infections.
- *Acne.* Common at puberty, usually unrelated to diet (a common myth).
- *Athlete's foot.* A fungal infection, commonly transmitted in locker-rooms or shower facilities.
- *Cradle cap.* A form of seborrhea, or dandruff. Mild redness and scaling or crusting patches on scalp or behind ears of young infants.
- *Chicken pox.* See earlier section in this chapter.
- *Measles.* Highly contagious viral disease causing a spreading red rash; rare now because of standard immunization.
- *Rubella* (German measles). Red rash caused by a mild viral infection, less contagious than measles, usually does not require treatment.
- *Roseola.* Caused by a viral infection that produces high fever and sometimes other symptoms before the rash appears; usually a mild disease, but is contagious.

In addition, rashes can be caused by the following five conditions.

Fifth Disease

Fifth disease is a contagious viral infection that usually causes no symptoms other than the rash (**Figure 13-6**). For most children it is a mild disease without complications and with no need for treatment. It can present a risk, however, to pregnant women or children with certain chronic illness.

When You See

- Bright red rash usually beginning on cheeks ("slapped cheek" appearance), later spreading to arms and legs

Do This First

1. Watch the child for other symptoms.
2. Try to prevent the infection spreading through direct contact.

Additional Care

Actions for parents:

- Monitor the child and take his or her temperature often; see a healthcare provider if fever or other symptoms occur.
- The child need not stay home.

Impetigo

Impetigo is a skin infection by streptococcal or other bacteria (**Figure 13-7**). The child feels very itchy and may scratch the area, then transmitting the infection to other body areas. It is easily transmitted to other children as well. Usually the infection is harmless, but a rare complication can cause a kidney problem (glomerulonephritis).

When You See

- Small red spots that progress to blisters that ooze and produce yellow-brown crusts
- Itchiness

Do This First

1. Prevent the child from scratching; child should wash hands often.
2. Wash and soak the area with soap and warm water to remove the crusts.
3. Follow your center's policy to apply a topical antibiotic ointment.
4. Prevent direct contact with others.

Additional Care

- Monitor the child for any other symptoms and healing of the rash within a few days.

Actions for parents:

- Call a healthcare provider if the rash does not improve in a few days, if the child has any other symptoms, or if the child's urine turns dark brown.
- The child can return to school or childcare a day after beginning to use the antibiotic ointment.

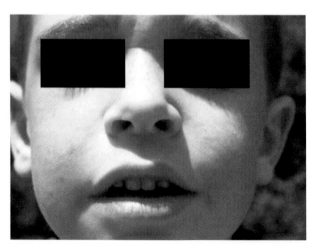

Figure 13-6 Fifth disease.

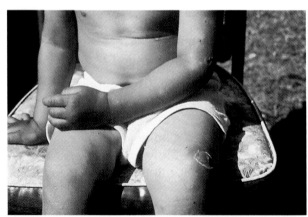

Figure 13-7 Impetigo.

Ringworm

Ringworm is a contagious fungal infection (and has nothing to do with worms). It spreads by direct contact. Ringworm can usually be treated with appropriate over-the-counter products (**Figure 13-8**).

When You See

- Rash begins as small round red spots that grow and become ring-shaped, with the ring border red, raised, and scaly.
- If the scalp is involved (rare), hair may fall out temporarily.

Do This First

1. Keep child from touching the area; avoid direct contact with others.
2. Wearing gloves, apply an antifungal ointment intended for ringworm (follow your center's policies).
3. Have child wash hands frequently.

Additional Care

Actions for parents:

- See a healthcare provider if the ringworm shows no improvement or keeps spreading after a week of treatment.
- While being treated, the child can attend school or childcare.

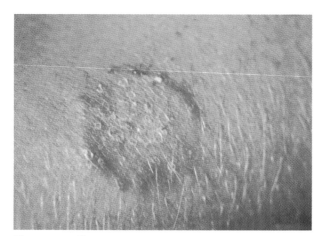

Figure 13-8 Ringworm.

Scabies

Scabies is a skin condition caused by tiny mites, related to chiggers, that dig into the skin and cause red bumps and severe itching (**Figure 13-9**). Typically the knee and elbow creases, armpits, and webbing between toes and fingers are affected. The infestation spreads by direct contact or indirect contact with a person's infested clothing. The child is likely to scratch the areas, which may then become infected.

When You See

- Severe itching
- Red bumps that may become oozing sores or blisters

Do This First

1. Give cool baths and use compresses or calamine to sooth itching.
2. The child needs to see a healthcare provider for a prescription anti-mite medication.

Additional Care

Actions for parents:

- All the child's bedding and clothing, including coats and hats, should be washed in hot water and dried on high heat. Use a hot dryer for stuffed toys, pillows, and cushions.
- Vacuum and clean all items and areas with which the child had contact in a childcare center, in the home, and in the family car. Anything that cannot be cleaned or heated in a clothes dryer should be sealed for 2 weeks in plastic bags.

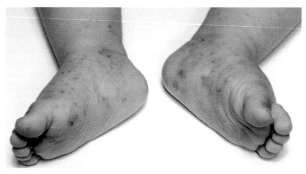

Figure 13-9 Scabies.

- Follow the healthcare provider's instructions for treatment with prescription ointment.
- One day after beginning the treatment, the child can return to school or childcare.

Scarlet Fever

Scarlet fever is caused by a streptococcal infection. Fever and fatigue often occur before the rash, along with headache, nausea, and vomiting. About 12 to 48 hours later the rash begins on the face, trunk, and arms and spreads to cover much of the body. The infection is contagious and spreads by direct contact or indirect contact when the victim sneezes (**Figure 13-10**).

When You See

- Intense red rash of tiny bumps lasting 5 days or more; skin then peels
- Tongue first has a white coating, and then turns red and swollen
- Red throat, and red spots on roof of mouth
- Sore throat

Do This First

1. Have child drink lots of fluids.
2. Follow your center's policy for giving children's acetaminophen or ibuprofen for high fever (parental permission required).

3. Prevent contact with other children, and encourage child to wash hands often.

Additional Care

Actions for parents:

- Take the child to a healthcare provider (an antibiotic will be prescribed).
- The child may return to school or childcare 1 day after starting the antibiotic, if fever has passed.

HEAD LICE

Head lice can occur on any child and are highly contagious. They spread by direct contact or through sharing hats, hairbrushes, or even coats touching when hung together (**Figure 13-11**).

When You See

- Frequent scratching of head
- Child complains of scalp itching
- Pinpoint red marks on scalp
- Tiny clusters of eggs (nits) like white lumps on hair

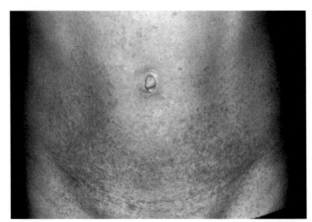

Figure 13-10 Scarlet fever.

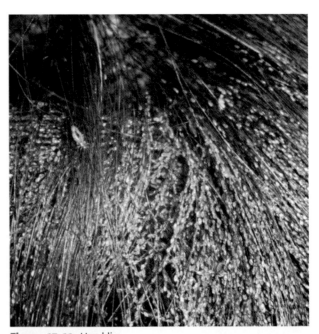

Figure 13-11 Head lice.

Do This First

1. Parents should use over-the-counter head lice shampoo, carefully following the product's directions; some products require multiple applications.

2. Family members, playmates, and others in contact with the child must be carefully checked for nits or signs of lice; all should be treated at the same time.

Additional Care

Actions for parents:

- All the child's bedding and clothing, including coats and hats, should be washed in hot water and dried on high heat. Use a hot dryer for stuffed toys, pillows, and cushions.

- Vacuum and clean all items and areas with which the child had contact in a childcare center, in the home, and in the family car. Anything that cannot be cleaned or heated in a clothes dryer should be sealed for 2 weeks in plastic bags.

- The child can return to school or childcare after completing treatment for head lice, following the site's specific policy.

Head Lice

Do not use lice shampoo on an infant. Wear gloves when using lice shampoo.

14 Preventing Infection and Illness

Earlier chapters have described care to give for most injuries and common illnesses that afflict children. It is just as important to work to prevent illness and injury from occurring in the first place. Most childhood injuries can in fact be prevented, as can many illnesses, by following accepted guidelines. These should be practiced in the home, in childcare, and in schools.

The following two chapters focus on preventing injury. This chapter describes measures all adults can take to help children stay healthy and avoid illness both now while they are children and, by starting healthy habits, into adulthood.

PREVENTING COMMON INFECTIONS

As you saw in the descriptions of common childhood illnesses in Chapter 13, many childhood illnesses are infectious: a child "catches" the disease from another child. Fortunately, vaccines and public health measures now prevent many of the serious infectious diseases of the past, and most childhood infectious illnesses are not life threatening.

Nonetheless, children are still frequently sick—averaging half a dozen illnesses a year until they reach school age, and then gradually diminishing. Most of these illnesses are infections caused by bacteria, viruses, fungi, or parasites.

Preventing children from catching or spreading infectious disease is based on understanding how disease is transmitted. This process involves four stages.

1. **The process begins with someone who has the infection.** In settings such as childcare centers, schools, or public places, children will eventually encounter someone who has an infectious disease.

2. **The infectious pathogen (bacteria, virus, fungus, or parasite) leaves the sick person's body.** Germs typically are present in some body fluid. When that fluid leaves the infected person's body, the germ may leave with it and enter the environment. For example:

- The person may sneeze out little droplets carrying the cold virus or tuberculosis bacteria.

- The person may bleed from a cut, and in that person's blood is the hepatitis A virus.

- The person may have a bowel movement and not wash his or her hands after wiping, thereby getting bacteria on the hands.

- Parasites on the person's scalp may crawl into his or her hat.

3. **The infectious pathogen reaches another child and enters his or her body. This can happen in a number of ways:**

   - The child may inhale the pathogen in tiny droplets in the air (**airborne transmission**).
   - The child may get a scrape, letting a pathogen from another person's blood get into his or her own blood (**bloodborne transmission**).
   - The child may be bitten by a tick or mosquito carrying the pathogen (**vector transmission**).
   - The child may touch the infected person (**direct contact**)**,** and the pathogen may pass directly from one to the other, as may happen with some infectious rashes or a fungus like ringworm.
   - The child may touch an object on which a pathogen is living after that object was in contact with the infected person (**indirect contact**)**.**
   - Once the child has a pathogen on his or her hands, it may enter the body when the child eats with his or her hands or wipes his or her eyes or mouth with the hands.

4. **The child develops the infection.** Just having the pathogen enter a child's body does not automatically mean he or she will become ill, however. The child may have been vaccinated against the disease, which means his or her body will kill the infection before it can cause the disease. The child may be very healthy and have a strong immune system that can kill a small amount of the pathogen and thereby prevent illness. Or the child may become sick—and then starts the process all over again with other children.

Preventing infection, therefore, involves stopping the spread of the pathogen by interrupting this process at any of the four stages:

1. If a sick person is not present, the disease cannot be transmitted. Childcare centers and schools therefore ask parents of children with many infectious diseases to keep their children home until they are no longer infectious. If you work in a childcare center, follow its policies for instructing parents when to keep their children home.

2. There is little you can do to prevent a pathogen from leaving an infected child's body—you cannot prevent a child from coughing or sneezing—but good hygiene practices can help prevent the pathogen from getting very far. Children can be taught to cover their mouths when they cough, to use tissues when they sneeze and dispose of the tissue correctly afterwards, and to wash their hands after toileting.

3. Most preventive measures focus on keeping the pathogen from reaching or entering a second child after it has left the first. All children should wash their hands, for example, before eating; this will help prevent a pathogen picked up by direct or indirect transmission from entering the child through the mouth. Wearing gloves when potentially contacting a child's body fluids also helps prevent transmission. Cleaning and disinfecting surfaces, eating and cooking utensils, and play areas also kills pathogens in the environment before they can reach and enter another child.

4. There is less that you as a caregiver can do to prevent illness if a pathogen does enter a child's body, but general preventive practices are still important. Parents need to make sure their children have all standard childhood vaccinations (see later section on immunization), which prevent most serious childhood diseases. Encouraging children to stay healthy by promoting a good diet, exercise, and appropriate weight also helps children stay strong so that their bodies fight diseases better. You may not be able to prevent the common cold by maintaining good health overall, but a generally healthy person's cold may not last as long or be as troublesome as it would if the person were in a state of poor health.

The following sections describe specific practices that help prevent transmission of infections in any group setting. If you work in a childcare center or school, your organization also has specific policies about actions you must take to help prevent infection.

Handwashing and Hygiene

Frequent good handwashing by both caregivers and children is the most important way to keep an infection from spreading. Follow these guidelines (**Figure 14-1**):

1. Wash frequently, and always in these situations (even if you were wearing gloves):

   - After any contact with a child known to have an infection
   - After any contact with body fluids (wear gloves)
   - After using the bathroom or changing a diaper (wear gloves)
   - Before touching food or eating
   - After outdoor activities

2. Use a good liquid soap. Your childcare center has likely chosen an effective type, such as an antibacterial hand soap.

3. Use warm water.

4. Rub your hands together and scrub everywhere up to the wrist. Interlace your fingers and rub them together. Scrub under the nails with a brush or nail stick.

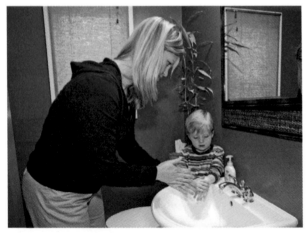

Figure 14-1 Handwashing is important for preventing the spread of infections.

5. Rinse your hands well and dry thoroughly with paper towels.

In addition to frequently washing your hands, practice good personal hygiene and teach children to do the same:

- Keep your hands away from your face, except when eating after having washed your hands. Do not smoke, apply makeup on the job, bite your nails, rub your nose, and so on.
- Use a tissue when sneezing. Cover your mouth when coughing.
- Properly dispose of used tissues and disposable gloves where others will not contact them.
- Keep your things clean and away from other people. These include cups or dishes, your toothbrush, and other personal items such as hairbrushes or your purse. Do not share personal things with others.

Cleaning and Disinfecting Areas

Cleaning means washing with soap and water, whereas disinfecting means killing all germs on an object or surface that may be contaminated with pathogens. Disinfection can be done with a commercial product or a 10% mixture of chlorine bleach in water. Any object or surface on which pathogens may be present or which potentially come into contact with body fluids should be regularly disinfected. Disinfect these objects and surfaces daily or after each use as appropriate:

- Toilets and potty seats
- Changing tables or areas
- Work tables
- Sinks
- Food preparation counters, equipment, and utensils
- Toys children put in their mouths, especially infant toys
- Any surface soiled by a body fluid
- Door knobs, toy cabinets, and other areas frequently touched by children

Soiled clothing or children's personal items that cannot be disinfected should be bagged and sealed for the parents to take home. Keep other children away from such items.

Areas not requiring daily disinfection should be cleaned daily or as needed, including such things as floors, wading pools, and outside toys.

Food Preparation

Follow these guidelines when preparing food or snacks for children:

- Wash dishes and utensils in a hot water commercial dishwasher if available, or rinse dishes in disinfectant solution before the final rinse with water.
- Remove jewelry such as bracelets and wash your hands before touching food, utensils, or surfaces, and wash again after touching meat.
- Do not prepare food or handle utensils if you may have an infectious illness.
- Keep long hair tied back or wear a hairnet, cap, or visor following state or local regulations.

- Keep diapers, used tissues, and other potentially contaminated things completely out of food preparation and eating areas.
- Make sure all children wash their hands before eating.

Immunizations

Vaccines prevent children from getting many serious infectious diseases. Pediatricians in the United States generally follow the immunization schedule approved by the Advisory Committee on Immunization Practices, the American Academy of Pediatrics, and the American Academy of Family Physicians. Children who receive these vaccines on the recommended schedule should be immune to these diseases (**Figure 14-2**):

- Diphtheria
- *H. influenzae* Type b (bacteria that causes meningitis and other disease)

Recommended Childhood and Adolescent Immunization Schedule
United States—June 2006

| Range of recommended ages | | | Catch-up immunization | | | 11–12 year old assessment | | | | | | | |

Vaccine / Age	Birth	1 month	2 months	4 months	6 months	12 months	15 months	18 months	24 months	4–6 years	11–12 years	13–14 years	15 years	16–18 years
Hepatitis B	HepB	HepB		HepB		HepB				HepB series				
Diphtheria, Tetanus, Pertussis			DTaP	DTaP	DTaP		DTaP			DTaP	Tdap	Tdap		
Haemophilus influenzae Type b			Hib	Hib	Hib	Hib								
Inactivated Poliovirus			IPV	IPV		IPV				IPV				
Measles, Mumps, Rubella						MMR				MMR		MMR		
Varicella						Varicella				Varicella				
Meningococcal							Vaccines within broken line are for selected populations		MPSV4		MCV4	MCV4 / MCV4		
Pneumococcal			PCV	PCV	PCV	PCV				PCV	PPV			
Influenza					Influenza (yearly)					Influenza (yearly)				
Hepatitis A								Hepatitis A series						

Figure 14-2 The recommended childhood immunization schedule.

- Hepatitis B
- Measles
- Meningococcus
- Mumps
- Pertussis (whooping cough)
- Polio
- Rubella (German measles)
- Tetanus
- Varicella (chicken pox)

For various reasons, however, not all children have had all these vaccinations or are current with boosters. Some states or school districts require vaccinations for children. Encourage parents to ensure their children have all recommended vaccinations.

Adult caregivers should consider their own vaccination status as well. A tetanus booster is generally recommended every 5 to 10 years. Many adults have not been vaccinated for hepatitis B, a serious disease caused by a bloodborne virus, and should consider getting this vaccination. An annual flu shot is also recommended for many adults who are exposed to a variety of people in their work. If you are employed in childcare, talk to your supervisor about recommended or required vaccinations.

WELL CHILD VISITS

Examinations of a healthy child by a pediatrician are called well child visits. These are recommended for ensuring not only the child's general health and immunizations but also to monitor growth and development and to detect potential problems early.

Well baby visits typically begin within 2 weeks of birth and include at least three more visits in the first year and two in the second. Thereafter, it is recommended that the child sees the pediatrician at least every year or two, with examinations recommended at ages 5, 6, 8, 10, 11, and 12. Public school systems often require examinations at specified ages or grades.

Following are some of the important screenings and examinations that take place at well child visits:

- Immunizations on the recommended schedule

- Measurements of height, weight, and head circumference (in an infant) to ensure normal growth and good nutrition
- A full physical examination to detect any abnormalities
- Blood pressure check
- Simple eye examination (with referral to an eye doctor in cases of vision problems)
- Hearing screening if a hearing disturbance is suspected
- Simple examination of developing teeth (with referral to a dentist if a problem is found)
- Discussion with parents and child about personal hygiene, diet, exercise, sleep, and emotional and mental health

Although childcare workers, teachers, and others without direct responsibility for the child's health are not usually involved in well child visits, they can encourage parents to promote their child's health in this way. When appropriate, childcare providers may suggest topics for parents to discuss with their child's healthcare provider at their next visit. Too often parents view healthcare providers as a resource only in times of illness, but well child visits can have an active role in promoting good health habits for life.

DENTAL CARE

An infant's first teeth usually appear at about 8 months but may be as early as 4 months or as late as 15. Teething can begin a month or more before the teeth appear. Teething can cause discomfort or pain. The child should be allowed to teeth on an appropriate hard rubber object but never on a bottle of milk, which can cause early decay or ear infections if the child is lying down.

Children can begin brushing their teeth as early as age 1 or 2 but typically are not proficient before about age four, and a child may need help brushing for several years after this (**Figure 14-3**). Children should be taught to brush their teeth within 5 to 10 minutes after eating. Regular brushing with a soft-bristle brush and fluoride toothpaste is recommended. Once-a-day flossing should begin with the permanent teeth,

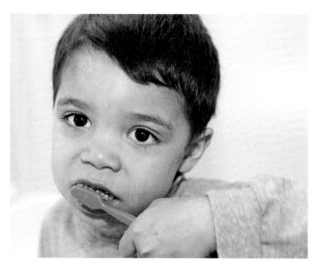

Figure 14-3. Even a toddler can start learning to brush his teeth, although he may not be proficient at it for several years.

which begin to erupt in the fifth or sixth year, to help prevent gum disease.

Loss of baby teeth is usually a natural process. Children typically wiggle loose teeth with their fingers or tongue until they come out on their own. Occasionally a very loose tooth that does not come out makes eating difficult. If the child wants, the parent may remove it by holding it with a piece of gauze and giving it a twist.

Regular dental examinations are recommended from about age 4 and at least annually thereafter, with most pediatricians and dentists recommending visits twice a year for cleaning and examination. Cavities may develop as early as age 3, however, but parents or caregivers can usually see cavities developing in the baby teeth. If so, even a young child should see a dentist. Early loss of or damage to baby teeth can cause pain or later dental problems with the permanent teeth, so parents and caregivers should attend to the child's teeth throughout early childhood and be alert for any problems. In areas where the water supply is not fluoridated, supplemental fluoride drops are often recommended for older infants and children.

Even though contemporary methods of applying sealants to permanent teeth have greatly helped reduce cavities in children, there is still need for brushing and flossing for complete dental health.

Remember that a tooth, even a baby tooth, that is knocked out in play or an injury may be reimplanted if the tooth is cared for and the child sees a dentist immediately. See the section on a knocked-out tooth in Chapter 3.

HABITS FOR A HEALTHY HEART

Most people know that heart disease is the major cause of death among adults, but fewer parents and caregivers understand that habits begun in early childhood lay the groundwork for the person's later cardiovascular health. Fortunately, in recent years more media attention has been given to the cardiovascular health of children. The problems of childhood obesity, high cholesterol levels, poor diet, and lack of exercise are now recognized. Although few children actually experience heart disease other than rare congenital problems, from a very early age they form habits that may stay with them for life—and could lead to a life shorter than it need be.

Diet, exercise, and weight control are crucial for maintaining a healthy heart. In addition, smoking contributes to poor cardiovascular health. Children learn about smoking at a very early age by observing adults. Do not smoke around children, both because of the risks of secondhand smoke and because you as an adult caregiver are a role model and are implicitly teaching the child it is okay to smoke. Support the efforts of schools and other organizations to teach children that all tobacco use is unhealthful.

Diet

Good nutrition affects the child's health right now as well as influencing habits that will affect cardiovascular health later on. Children's food preferences are influenced by many factors, such as what the family eats at home, what they see other children eat at childcare or at school, and what television commercials "teach" them to eat. You cannot counteract all these influences, of course, but encouraging a good diet is the responsibility of all adult caregivers.

Most current nutritional research continues to support what we have known for some time: high-fat and high-sugar foods are unhealthy, and eating a variety of foods with an emphasis on fruits, vegetables, and whole grains and cereals is healthy and promotes a normal weight. Follow these guidelines if you are involved with feeding children or when talking with parents about what their children eat:

- Minimize sweets. Encourage fruit rather than candy, and juice rather than sodas.
- Minimize high-fat and high-cholesterol foods, such as potato chips and many fast foods.
- Follow the food guide pyramid, which emphasizes grains and cereals, followed by fruits and vegetables, with lesser amounts of dairy products, and only sparing use of fats, oils, and sweets.
- Eat a variety of foods rather than habitually only a few.
- Watch portion size. The phenomenon of "supersizing" food portions has led many people to consume more at a meal or snack than they need to feel full.
- Choose high-fiber foods rather than refined foods (whole grains rather than white flour products, plus fruits and vegetables).
- Choose lean meats rather than fatty ones, and cut away visible fat and chicken skin.
- Minimize fried foods (such as french fries, fried chicken, doughnuts).
- Choose low-salt foods (heavy use of salt becomes a habit that will likely persist into adulthood and may contribute to high blood pressure).

In almost all instances, healthy alternatives to unhealthy foods and snacks are available that taste just as good. Children like low-fat frozen yogurt or frozen fruit bars as much as ice cream, low-fat milk as much as whole milk, whole wheat bread as much as white bread, and so on. In all these ways you will help set the stage for a lifetime of cardiovascular health.

Exercise

It has become a cliché but is nonetheless true: Most children do not get enough exercise. Television, computer games, and the Internet have

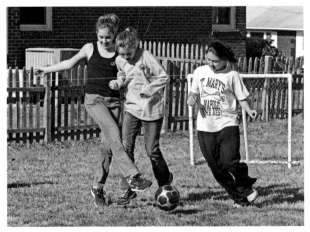

Figure 14-4 Exercise and physical activity promote good health.

contributed to children becoming more sedentary than decades ago. Exercise is good not only for the muscles but also for the heart, lungs, and blood vessels. Like diet, exercise helps a child be healthier now and builds a foundation for future cardiovascular health and a longer, healthier, happier life. As a caregiver you can help promote exercise and physical activity (**Figure 14-4**).

- Children need to exercise moderately strenuously three to five times a week for at least 20 to 30 minutes.
- Children will get more exercise if it is fun. Almost all age-appropriate sports and energetic activities that children enjoy are good forms of cardiovascular exercise. Even brisk walking counts.
- Make physical activity a routine part of the day, not a special requirement at certain times. Help children think of physical activity as being as "normal" in their life as eating or sleeping.
- Childcare providers have many opportunities to help children stay physically active. If you are employed in a childcare center, participate in your center's activities that provide adequate exercise, and talk with your supervisor about other ideas to help children be active.

Maintaining a Healthy Weight

A child who eats well and gets exercise is unlikely to become overweight. Yet in America today, according to some estimates, more than one-quarter of children are overweight and many of those are obese. Overweight and obesity contribute to many adult diseases in addition to heart disease, and the habits that lead to overweight start early in a child's life. Prevention is a better approach than having to lose weight later on and keep it off.

Follow the earlier recommendations for diet and exercise to promote children's health and an appropriate weight. Be sensitive to the feelings of parents of overweight children, however, for eating and weight issues involve many psychological factors. Encourage well child visits, where the pediatrician will determine the child's appropriate weight and help the family develop a weight loss plan that will work for them.

15 Preventing Injuries

Children, especially young children, are at risk for injury because they are naturally active and fearlessly explore their environment. They will touch almost anything or put it in their mouths. They will climb on things, pull on things, fall off things, put their heads in things. Since it is impossible to monitor all children at all times in all settings, childcare providers and parents must take steps to prevent injuries such as choking, poisoning, burns, and traumatic injury.

PREVENTING CHOKING

Choking is a serious threat to infants and children up to 3 or 4 years of age and a major cause of death. An infant or young child may put any small object in his or her mouth, but food causes most cases of choking (**Figure 15-1**). Follow these guidelines to prevent choking:

• Do not leave any small objects within reach of an infant (such as buttons, beads, coins). Ensure that small parts cannot break off toys or other items around the infant or young child.
• Feed infants only soft foods that do not require chewing.
• Have children sit in a high chair or at a table to eat. Never let a child move around while eating.
• Teach children not to eat too fast or to talk or laugh while eating.

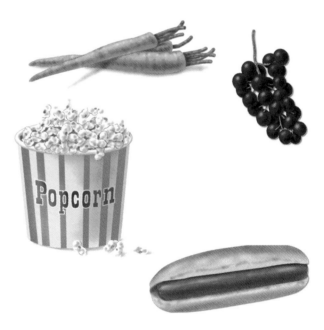

Figure 15-1 Do not give a child under age 3 any foods that could cause choking.

- Cut up foods in very small pieces, especially foods a child could choke on, such as hot dogs.
- Do not give children under age 3 these foods:
  - Peanuts
  - Popcorn
  - Grapes
  - Chunks of raw vegetables or fruits
  - Marshmallows
  - Gum
- Supervise young children while they eat, and be prepared to care for a child who chokes (see Chapter 2).

PREVENTING POISONING

Most childhood poisonings happen in the home, but a poisoning can happen anywhere children are present. Household products such as cleaning supplies and plants are the two most common poisons, followed by medicines, other chemicals and products, insecticides and pesticides, and adhesives and glues. Improper use of medications, such as accidentally giving a young child an adult dose of acetaminophen, also causes many poisonings.

Preventing poisoning begins with safe storage of all substances that could potentially poison a child:

- Keep all cleaning and other liquid or solid products away from children. Keep them in special storage cabinets with childproof latches or locks, or on high shelves (**Figure 15-2**).

- Read all product labels to determine what may be poisonous to a child. Personal hygiene products in a bathroom, for example, may be poisons and should be stored elsewhere.
- With all potentially poisonous products, choose brands with childproof caps—even if you plan to store the product in a locked cabinet.
- Keep all products in their original containers for safe use and because if a poisoning does occur, you will need to know the product's ingredients.
- Teach children about poison symbols and to stay away when they see them.
- Lock areas such as a shed or garage where lawn and garden chemicals and other poisonous products are kept, even if you think a child would never go there.
- Get on your hands and knees and check all areas where children may go, looking for *anything* they might put in their mouth.
- Check the labels of products, such as paints and glues, used in arts and crafts projects.
- Remember to watch for poisons in other places where you take children.

Remember that many houseplants as well as plants found in gardens or parks are also poisonous. Rather than trying to memorize several dozens of common plants that are poisonous, it is safest to keep *all* houseplants out of children's reach. This includes plants, boughs,

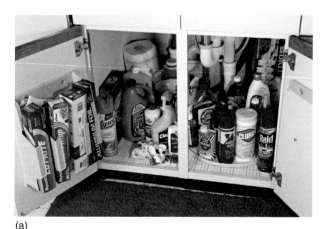
(a)

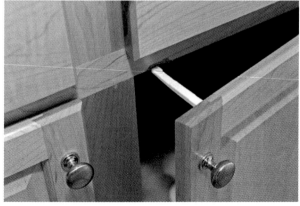
(b)

Figure 15-2 Many household products are poisons and should be kept in cabinets that are locked (a) or have childproof latches (b).

flowers, and berries often used for holiday decorations. Outdoors, there is no substitute for close supervision to make sure young children do not put flowers, berries, or leaves in their mouths.

Also take special care with both prescription and nonprescription medications:

- Never refer to a medicine as candy to entice a child to take it. The child may come back for more.
- Use childproof safety caps. Store the medicines in a locked or childproofed cabinet.
- Always check the dosage on the label before giving a medication, even if you are sure you remember it.
- Do not give anyone's medication to someone else.
- Properly dispose of outdated products.

Almost all accidental poisonings can be prevented, but stay prepared in case one does occur:

- Remember the first aid for poisoning and to call the Poison Control Center (see Chapter 9). Take the number with you if you carry a cell phone on outings with children. The toll-free national number is 1-800-222-1222.
- Keep activated charcoal in your first aid kit, but remember it is not always used. Use it only if the Poison Control Center tells you to do so for a specific poison.

Preventing Carbon Monoxide Poisoning

Carbon monoxide is an odorless poisonous gas produced by the incomplete burning of fuels. To prevent carbon monoxide poisoning, follow these guidelines:

- Have your building's heating system, chimneys, and flues inspected and cleaned or repaired as needed.
- Be sure the furnace has good intake of fresh air.
- Be sure the flue is open when fireplace is used.
- Do not use a gas stove or oven to heat an area.

- Never burn charcoal indoors.
- Do not use unvented gas or kerosene heaters in an enclosed area.

PREVENTING BURNS

Preventing burns in children involves both preventing fires and preventing burns from hot water and objects such as stoves.

Preventing Fires

Follow these guidelines to prevent a fire in a childcare center or home (**Figure 15-3**):

- Electricity often causes fires. Keep power cords away from children.
- Store matches, lighters, candles, and other ignition sources away from children.
- Check appliance cords for damaged areas or fraying.
- Keep cords away from counter edges where children may pull on them.
- Do not overload electrical outlets or use multiple extension cords.
- Make sure enough smoke detectors are installed and have good batteries (change batteries twice a year when you change your clocks for daylight savings time).
- Make sure there are fire extinguishers in cooking areas, and know how to use them.
- Tie back long hair or loose clothing when cooking or working around flames.
- Plan escape routes and hold regular fire drills with children. Post escape routes in a prominent place. Teach children to "stop, drop, and roll" if their clothing catches on fire.
- Do not allow smoking anywhere in the building.
- Keep curtains and other flammable objects away from fireplaces and stoves.
- Have chimneys inspected and cleaned to prevent chimney fires.
- Never store gasoline or other highly flammable liquids indoors.
- Unplug appliances when not in use.

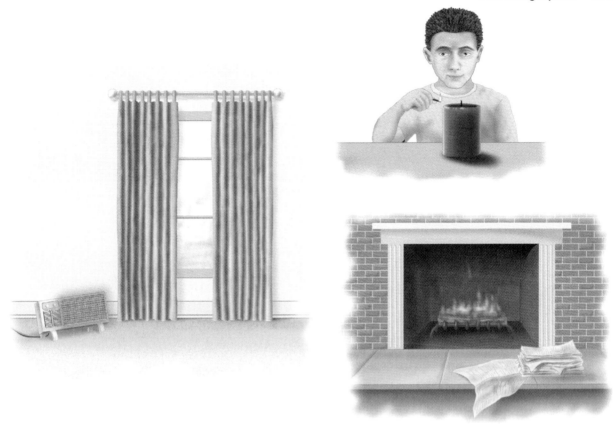

Figure 15-3 Inspect all rooms for fire hazards, and keep children away from flames and sources of heat.

If a Fire Happens

Because a fire may occur even when you try to prevent it, know what to do if one should break out:

- Evacuate everyone and call 9-1-1 first. Do not delay evacuation while you use a fire extinguisher. Follow the rehearsed evacuation route.
- Do not use an elevator.
- Feel doors before opening them, and do not open a door that is hot.
- If the air is smoky, stay near the floor where there is more oxygen.
- Do not throw water on an electrical or grease (cooking) fire.
- If food catches on fire in a microwave or toaster oven, leave the food there and turn the appliance off; keep other objects away until the flames go out.
- Stop, drop, and roll if your clothing catches on fire.

- If you cannot escape a building on fire, stuff clothing or rags in door cracks and vents; call 9-1-1 and give the dispatcher your exact location.

Preventing Heat Burns

- Prevent scalding burns by turning down the temperature of the water heater to 120 degrees Fahrenheit or lower (state regulations may apply in childcare centers).
- Supervise children in the bathtub.
- When cooking, use back burners and keep pot handles turned toward the back of the stove.
- Do not store food near the stove because children may attempt to reach it on their own.
- Keep hot irons away from children (**Figure 15-4**).
- Do not use steam vaporizers, or keep them away from areas children can reach.

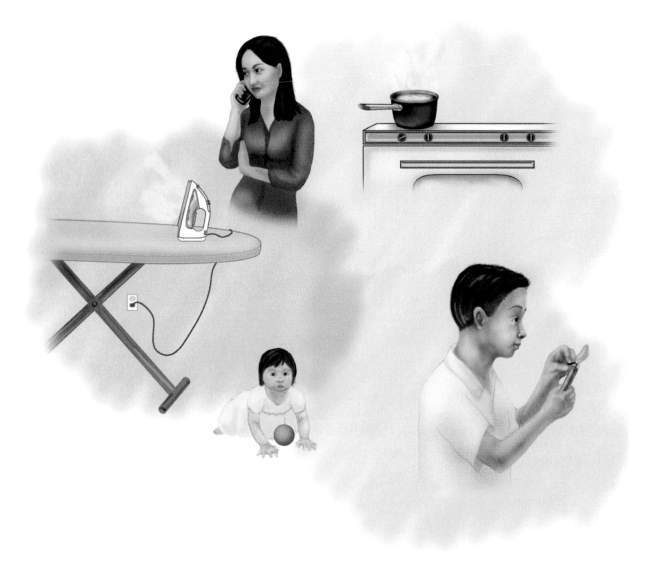

Figure 15-4 Children need to be protected from many sources of heat.

- Do not use space heaters on the floor or anywhere children can reach them.
- Never let children use fireworks.
- Prevent sunburn:
  - Use frequent applications of a sunscreen with a sun protection factor (SPF) of 30 or higher on all exposed areas of skin (**Figure 15-5**).
  - Keep infants and young children covered with light clothing and hats.
  - Limit sun exposure from 10 o'clock a.m. to 4 o'clock p.m.
  - Be aware that reflective surfaces like water and snow increase the risk of burning.

Remember the first aid for a child who is burned (see Chapter 5).

PREVENTING ELECTRICAL SHOCK

Electricity may cause life-threatening shocks as well as electrical burns. Follow these guidelines to keep children safe (**Figure 15-6**):

- Use outlet caps to block unused electrical outlets.
- Never use electrical appliances near water or when your hands are wet.
- Inspect electrical cords for broken or frayed insulation.

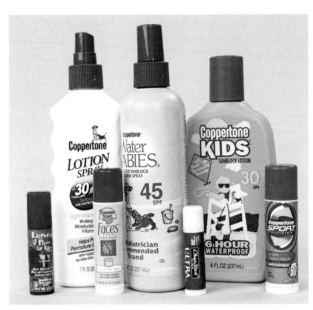

Figure 15-5 Protect against sunburn with frequent use of sunscreen.

- Be careful not to touch the wire prongs when inserting or removing plugs.
- Install a ground fault circuit interrupter (GFCI) in outlets in bathrooms and kitchens.
- When outdoors, keep everyone away from downed power lines, and do not let children play near electrical poles or fly kites near wires.

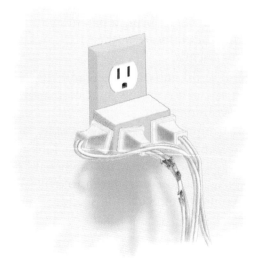

Figure 15-6 Overloaded outlets or extension cords pose a risk of fire or electrical shocks.

PREVENTING TRAUMATIC INJURY

In the United States traumatic injury is the leading cause of death in children, and over half a million children are hospitalized with serious injuries every year. The most common types of traumatic injury are motor vehicle passenger injuries, pedestrian injuries, bicycle injuries, and firearm injuries. Children are more susceptible to injury for several reasons:

- Children's heads are proportionally larger than adults, making head injury more likely.
- Children's senses are less developed than adults', making them more likely not to see or hear a danger coming (such as a car approaching when walking or riding a bike).
- Children are generally active and exploratory, often putting themselves into risky situations.
- Children have not learned about many dangers and when playing are usually preoccupied with other thoughts.

Most injuries can be prevented, however. Strategies for keeping children safe from injury involve three general principles:

1. Keep children away from dangers.
2. Stay near children and supervise their activity.
3. Teach children safety rules.

These general principles may seem common sense, but caregivers must diligently inspect and monitor every aspect of the child's environment to ensure no dangers are present (**Figure 15-7**). Chapter 16 describes things to check for both inside the building and outside and safety rules to teach children. In addition, keep a first aid kit handy and know the care to give if the child is injured.

PREVENTING VIOLENCE

Children are not immune to the violence in our society. Fortunately, in most childcare settings, violence is rare. Injuries caused by violent behavior of other children can generally be prevented with adequate adult supervision.

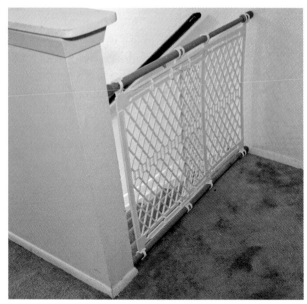

Figure 15-7 A childproof gate across the top of a stairway is a simple but effective way of keeping infants and toddlers away from danger.

When taking children on field trips or other excursions into public places, however, caregivers need to be especially vigilant. Vehicular traffic can be a threat to children as pedestrians, especially when crossing streets. Avoid taking children to crowded public places where it may be easy to lose sight of a child or where older children engaged in boisterous play may injure a young child. All communities have safe public places where children can play, and it is worth any needed extra effort to take children in your care to such places rather than risk their safety.

Preventing Abuse

Child abuse is another significant cause of traumatic injury to children. Although caretakers outside the home cannot directly prevent abuse within the child's home, they can—and should—act to prevent the continuation of abuse if they suspect it is occurring. Chapter 12

describes the signs of abuse and what to do if you see them. If you suspect a child is being abused or is at risk of being injured, you should report it and let the child protective services agency handle the situation.

Firearm Safety

Because many children are injured or killed every year by guns in the home, firearm safety should be a concern for all adults. Toy guns are common and often lead children to play with real guns if they find them in the home. Here is what you can do to help prevent the needless tragedy of children being injured by guns:

- If you have a gun in your own home, keep it locked up, with the ammunition in a separate locked cabinet. A trigger lock provides additional protection.
- Many experts argue children should not play with toy guns at all, but if you allow a child to have a toy gun, choose one whose appearance is not easily confused with a real gun. Teach children guns are dangerous. Many schools and centers have policies against "shooting" at other children even with a stick or finger.
- Teach children that if they encounter a gun in a friend's house or elsewhere, they must stay away from it or leave the house.
- Be alert for even very young children who may innocently bring a parent's gun to school or childcare in their backpack to show friends.
- Because BB guns, air rifles, and knives can also cause serious injuries, the same preventions apply.
- Firearm prevention applies to older children and teenagers as well, who may look for and find the key to a gun cabinet at home. Teenagers and even preteens often use guns to commit homicide and suicide.

16 Making Places Safe for Children

The previous chapter described general principles for preventing most childhood injuries. This chapter presents a series of checklists you can use to inspect your home, childcare center, and other settings to ensure all places are safe for children.

HOME AND CHILDCARE

Check all areas both inside and outside the building for safety.

Inside the Building

A good approach is to check each room one at a time for hazards (**Figure 16-1**).

Outside the Building

Garage and Storage Areas

- ❏ Garage and storage areas with garden chemicals and other products are always locked (**Figure 16-2**)?
- ❏ Tools and sharp objects are stored out of reach?
- ❏ Ropes and cords are stored out of reach?
- ❏ Trash is stored in secure containers?
- ❏ Areas are well lit and free of obstructions?

Yard

- ❏ Poisonous plants have been removed, and children are monitored to prevent eating any plants?
- ❏ Plants with thorns or scratch parts are pruned back? (To prevent scratches to child's eyes.)
- ❏ Pets are kept out of play areas?

- ❏ Fenced yards have childproof gates?
- ❏ No gardening tools or supplies are left out where children can reach them?
- ❏ Sandboxes and wading pools are covered between uses?
- ❏ All children are observed when playing in wading pools?
- ❏ Outdoor furniture and play equipment are sturdy and safe? Well anchored? On a soft surface?
- ❏ See also later section on playgrounds.
- ❏ See also next section on home pools.

Home Swimming Pools

- ❏ Is pool surrounded by a secure fence with childproof gate?
- ❏ Is a floating alarm used to detect someone falling in?
- ❏ Pool decking is nonskid?
- ❏ Children are always supervised? Allowed only in appropriate depths (not depending on inflatable toys)?
- ❏ Children are taught not to dive in water less than 9 feet deep?
- ❏ A barrier is present between shallow and deep water?

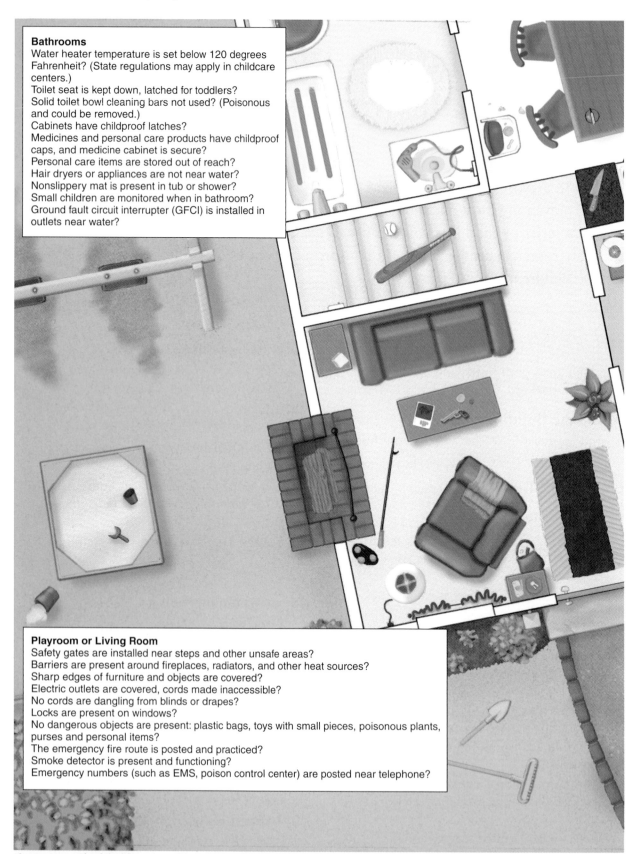

Bathrooms
Water heater temperature is set below 120 degrees Fahrenheit? (State regulations may apply in childcare centers.)
Toilet seat is kept down, latched for toddlers?
Solid toilet bowl cleaning bars not used? (Poisonous and could be removed.)
Cabinets have childproof latches?
Medicines and personal care products have childproof caps, and medicine cabinet is secure?
Personal care items are stored out of reach?
Hair dryers or appliances are not near water?
Nonslippery mat is present in tub or shower?
Small children are monitored when in bathroom?
Ground fault circuit interrupter (GFCI) is installed in outlets near water?

Playroom or Living Room
Safety gates are installed near steps and other unsafe areas?
Barriers are present around fireplaces, radiators, and other heat sources?
Sharp edges of furniture and objects are covered?
Electric outlets are covered, cords made inaccessible?
No cords are dangling from blinds or drapes?
Locks are present on windows?
No dangerous objects are present: plastic bags, toys with small pieces, poisonous plants, purses and personal items?
The emergency fire route is posted and practiced?
Smoke detector is present and functioning?
Emergency numbers (such as EMS, poison control center) are posted near telephone?

Figure 16-1 Check inside and outside the building for hazards.

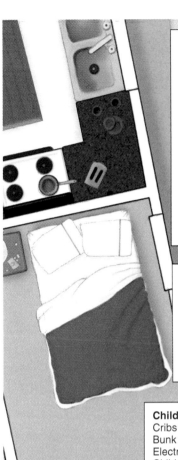

Kitchen and Laundry Area
Hot foods and liquids are kept from counter edges?
Stools and chairs are not near work counters? (Children may climb up.)
Meals are not left standing at room temperature? (Bacteria may grow.)
Knives and sharp objects are secured from children?
Appliance cords are secured out of children's reach?
No flammable objects are near stove or cooking appliances?
Childproof latches are present on lower cabinets?
Trash can is kept in a latched cabinet?
No cleaning or other products can be reached by children?
Pots on stove have handles turned to the rear?
Highchairs are placed well away from stove, appliances, telephone cord?
Smoke detector is present and functioning?
Tablecloth is not used? (Can be pulled off and drop objects on toddler.)
Refrigerator has childproof latch? "Sell by" dates on foods checked?
Children are taught to keep hands out of garbage disposal?
Washer and dryer doors are kept closed?

Hallways and Stairs
Walkways are clear?
Stairs and halls are well lit?
Safety gates are used at top and bottom of stairs?
Safety gates have top rail rather than open V-shape that could trap child's head?
Slippery throw rugs are not used, or nonskid mats are used?
Handrails and banisters are secure, and banister posts are no more than 4 inches apart?

Child's Bedroom or Sleeping Areas
Cribs and beds are far from radiators and other heat sources?
Bunk beds have safety rails? Children are not allowed to play on top bunk?
Electric cords are not within reach?
Children's sleepwear is flame resistant?
Toy box lid cannot fall down on children?
No small objects or toy parts are present?
Smoke detector is present and functioning?
Emergency fire route is rehearsed?
Infant's changing area:
• Floor pad is used for changing (safer than a table)?
• Changing supplies are kept at hand so infant is never left alone?
• Talcum power is not used, or if used, is sprinkled away from infant? (To prevent being inhaled.)

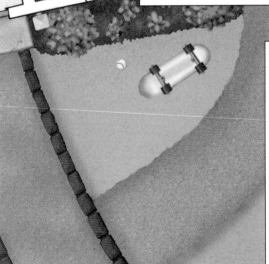

All Rooms
Barriers are present around fireplaces, radiators, and other heat sources?
Nontoxic paint is used on all surfaces (no lead paint)?
There are no tears in carpets or rugs that may cause tripping?
Cosmetics, personal items, and all flammable or breakable objects are kept out of children's reach?
Electric outlets are covered, cords secured?
Smoke detector and carbon monoxide detector (in appropriate areas) are present and functioning?
No cords dangle from blinds or drapes?
Latches are present on windows and used? There is no furniture under windows that children may climb up? Window guards (with emergency releases) or safety netting is installed on upstairs windows?
Doors to outside are kept latched?
Mothballs (poisonous) are not accessible in closets or storage boxes?

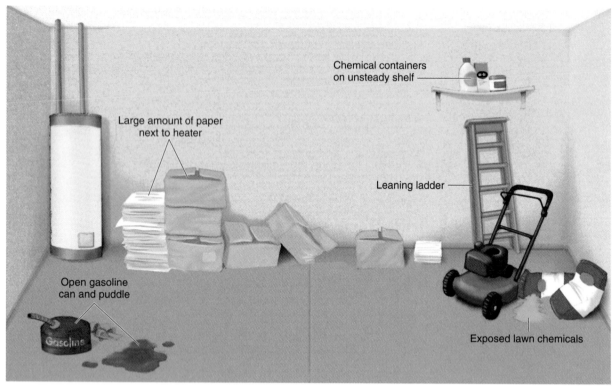

Figure 16-2 Garage and storage areas can be potentially hazardous.

☐ The outside ladder is removed from an above-ground pool when not in use?

☐ See also later section on water safety.

Pedestrian Safety

☐ Children are taught to stay on the sidewalk and out of the street?

☐ Children are taught to keep away from parked cars and trucks?

☐ Smaller children's hands are held to keep them from running off?

☐ Children are taught at appropriate age how to cross streets safely? (Use crosswalks, look left-right-left.)

Safety in Public Places

☐ Children are taught to stay away from strangers?

☐ Children are kept together in group so all can be watched?

EQUIPMENT FOR INFANTS AND TODDLERS

Cribs

☐ The crib design is safe and meets current standards (**Figure 16-3**)?

☐ The crib is deep enough to prevent child from climbing out?

☐ Spaces between bars and other openings are no more than $2^3/_8$ inches wide? (To prevent trapping head.)

☐ Corner posts are no more than $1/_{16}$ above height of sides? (To prevent catching clothing.)

☐ Latches on drop rail are secure and cannot be opened by child?

☐ The gap between mattress and crib sides is no more than 1½ inches? (To prevent trapping head.)

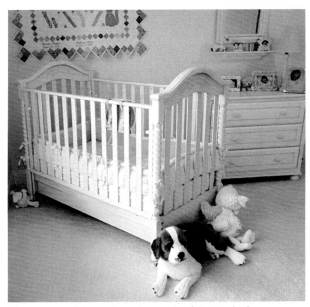

Figure 16-3 Crib must meet current safety standards.

❑ Plastic sheeting or bags is not used as mattress or pillow cover? (To prevent suffocation.)

❑ There is no rough wood or metal inside crib? No screws, bolts, or hardware loose or missing?

❑ A pillow is not used for an infant under 1 year? (To prevent suffocation.)

❑ Heavy comforters or blankets are not used? (To prevent suffocation.)

❑ Crib bumpers are removed when infant can sit up? (To prevent using them to climb out.)

❑ No toys other than small soft toys are present in crib?

❑ A cord is not used on a pacifier? (To prevent strangulation.)

❑ No cords with toys span the crib? (To prevent strangulation.)

❑ Infants not put to bed on their stomach? (A risk factor in sudden infant death.)

❑ The crib mattress is moved to its lowest position when the child can pull himself to standing position?

Play Yards (Playpens)

❑ Mesh holes are no bigger than ¼ inch?

❑ There is no rough wood or metal inside?

❑ There are no tears in mesh sides?

❑ Large toys are kept out of play yard? (Child could climb out.)

❑ The play yard is positioned where you can see children in it?

❑ The play yard is kept away from stove and counters where things could fall in?

❑ No cords with toys span the play yard? (To prevent strangulation.)

❑ Play yard is not used for children who can climb out or who are over 30 pounds?

High Chairs

❑ High chair is stable, with widely spaced legs?

❑ Tray is secure and cannot be moved by child?

❑ Safety harness (not just waist belt) is always used?

❑ Child is never left alone in highchair?

❑ High chair is positioned away from stove, counters, and telephone cords?

Strollers

❑ The design is stable and secure (**Figure 16-4**)?

❑ The stroller has large wheels for uneven surfaces and steps?

❑ The brakes lock both wheels? Brakes are used whenever stroller is parked?

❑ The safety harness is always used?

❑ The child is never left unattended in stroller?

❑ The stroller is not overloaded or top-heavy with equipment? (To prevent turning over.)

❑ Bags are not hung on the handles? (To prevent turning over.)

Baby Exercisers

❑ Baby walkers are not used? (Unsafe, easily turn over.)

❑ Baby exercisers such as Bouncers and ExerSaucers™ are used only for limited times? (Safer but may not promote child development.)

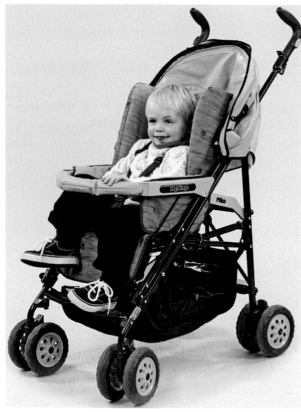

Figure 16-4 Strollers should meet safety standards.

- ❑ Push cars or wagons are sturdy and will not tip over?
- ❑ Children are always kept in view?

Baby Swings

- ❑ The swing has a wide base?
- ❑ The construction is sturdy and legs are secure?
- ❑ The safety harness is always used?
- ❑ The child is never left unattended?

RECREATIONAL SAFETY

Playground Safety

- ❑ The playground is fenced and away from roads (**Figure 16-5**)?
- ❑ Dogs are not allowed inside?
- ❑ Children play only on age-appropriate equipment?
- ❑ Toddler areas are apart from areas for older children?

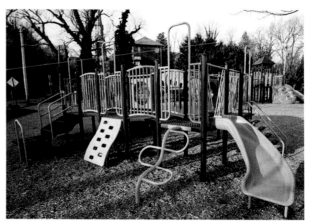

Figure 16-5 A safe playground area.

- ❑ All equipment is sturdy and stable, legs have wide bases and are anchored?
- ❑ Surfaces around equipment have 12 inches of loose fill (wood chips or mulch, sand, pea gravel, shredded rubber) or other soft padding?
- ❑ There are no exposed concrete footings, rocks, or objects that could cause tripping?
- ❑ There is a 6-foot open zone around stationary equipment?
- ❑ All openings in equipment (including guardrails and ladders) are less than 3½ or more than 9 inches wide? (To prevent trapping child's head or body.)
- ❑ Guardrails are present on elevated platforms, at least 29 inches high for preschoolers and 38 inches high for older children?
- ❑ Equipment is checked for wood splinters, sharp edges, protruding bolts, other dangerous hardware?
- ❑ Children's hoods, drawstrings, and other clothing that could become caught are removed?
- ❑ Children are always supervised?
- ❑ Specific equipment needs:
  - ❑ Swings have soft seats, at least 24 inches apart, away from other equipment? Toddlers use bucket seats?
  - ❑ Slides are well anchored, not higher than 8 feet; have handrails, nonslippery steps, and horizontal exit portion; are used by one child at a time, always sliding feet-first?

❏ Climbing structures are not used by children under age 4, have sturdy steps and handrails, and are supervised (many experts recommend avoiding monkey bars)?

❏ Merry-go-rounds have good hand grips, level rotating surface, and no sharp edges; and are close to ground to prevent crushing injuries?

Toy Safety

❏ Toys are checked for safety approval labels when purchased?

❏ Children play only with age-appropriate toys? (Manufacturer's recommendations plus common sense.)

❏ Secondhand toys without labels are never used? (Could be unsafe or have lead paint.)

❏ Toys are checked for sharp edges or protruding points (avoid thin plastic that easily breaks) and small parts that may break off? (Choking hazard.)

❏ Paints, crayons, craft supplies are nontoxic?

❏ Fresh batteries are not mixed with old ones? (Could cause overheating.)

❏ Uninflated or popped balloons are kept from small children? (Choking hazard.)

❏ Toy box lids are strong and cannot close unexpectedly?

❏ Cords are not used on pacifiers or toys for infants or small children? (Suffocation hazard.)

Bicycle Safety

❏ Children wear a helmet approved by the U.S. Consumer Product Safety Commission (CPSC) with chin strap that fits snugly (**Figure 16-6**)?

❏ Bicycles have safety equipment (reflectors front and rear and on pedals and spokes, horn or bell)? Right size for child? (Too big is unsafe.)

❏ Bicycles are inspected before use (nothing broken or loose, brakes adjusted, tires full)?

❏ Only children over age 11 are allowed to ride on streets with traffic?

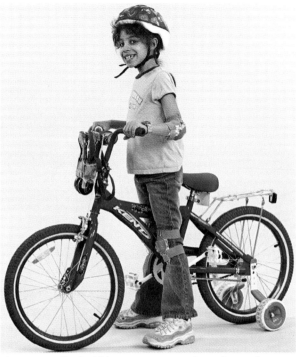

Figure 16-6 Teach children to wear appropriate safety equipment.

❏ Children are dressed in bright colors for visibility? Leg bands are used on baggy pant cuffs? No bare feet?

❏ Children are not allowed to ride at night?

❏ Children never wear earphones while riding?

❏ Children are taught bicycle safety rules?
  ❏ Ride single file with traffic not against it, staying to far right.
  ❏ Use hand signals before turning.
  ❏ Obey traffic signs and rules.
  ❏ Stop at all intersections and look left-right-left and over shoulder.
  ❏ Never hitch a ride on a motor vehicle.

❏ Adults use child carriers safely?
  ❏ Choose approved carrier with back higher than child's head, protections to keep child's feet from spokes, and a sturdy, secure harness.
  ❏ Both you and child should wear helmets.
  ❏ Compensate for added weight and longer braking times.

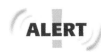

Skateboard and Inline Skates

❑ Children wear a CPSC-approved helmet
with chin strap that fits snugly?

❑ Safety gear is used (elbow and knee pads,
wrist guards, gloves)?

❑ Skates/skateboard is inspected before use
(nothing broken or loose, wheels or brakes
not worn)?

❑ Children learn to fall (relax body, roll on
impact, do not absorb force with arms)
using padded mats indoors or soft lawn
outdoors?

❑ Children learn on a level, smooth surface?

❑ Children learn to stop and practice this
skill?

❑ Children taught skating/boarding safety
rules?

    ❑ Stay out of streets and crowded
    pedestrian ways.

    ❑ Stay on the right side of paths.

    ❑ When passing a slower skater, pass on left
    after calling ahead: "Passing on left."

    ❑ Never hitch a ride from a motor vehicle
    or bicycle.

    ❑ Do not take chances trying tricks or
    jumps except with training in specially
    designed areas (homemade ramps are
    often dangerous).

    ❑ Follow traffic rules and yield to
    pedestrians.

Sledding Safety

❑ Sled or toboggan is in good condition with
no broken parts or sharp edges?

❑ Gentle hill with safe run-off is chosen for
sledding? (Not near frozen lake, pond, or
river.)

❑ Site is free of obstacles such as trees, traffic,
rocks, fences?

❑ Children are dressed warmly with thick gloves
and boots to prevent frostbite and injury? (See
later section on preventing cold injuries.)

Sports Safety

❑ Proper sports equipment is always used?

❑ Coaches are trained in first aid and know
not to overexert children?

❑ Playing fields or courts are checked for safe
conditions? Children cannot leave the area
into traffic or other hazards?

❑ Children stop playing when hurt or in pain?

❑ Measures are taken with older children in
team sports to prevent common injuries?

    ❑ Children play and compete with players
    of comparable size and development?

    ❑ Children train and do physical
    conditioning in preparation for sports?

    ❑ Overuse of arm and leg muscles is
    prevented?

    ❑ Children stretch and warm up before
    sports activities?

    ❑ Water breaks are taken about every 20
    minutes?

    ❑ Heat illnesses are prevented in hot weather
    by adequate breaks and hydration?

    ❑ Team has emergency plan in case of
    injuries?

    ❑ Children with health conditions see a
    healthcare provider before participating
    in sports?

Preventing Heat Emergencies

❑ Outdoor activities are limited when
temperatures rise?

❑ Activity breaks are taken often? Out of the
sun and heat?

❑ Children are given plenty of cold water to
drink?

❏ Children are dressed in light, loose clothing?

❏ Children are not left in hot vehicle or unventilated room?

❏ Wading pool or sprinkler is used to cool children?

Preventing Cold Emergencies

❏ Children are dressed for the cold (layers of loose-fitting, damp-resistant clothing; warm hats, gloves, and boots)?

❏ Face and neck are protected with scarf, turtleneck sweater, or face mask?

❏ Adult supervisors check children frequently for signs of becoming cold?

❏ Children stay indoors when wind chill makes exposure dangerous?

Avoiding Bites and Stings

Preventing Tick Bites

❏ Pant legs are tucked into socks or boots when in tick areas, or rubber-banded against socks?

❏ Shirts are tucked into pants?

❏ Light clothing is worn to make it easier to see ticks?

❏ Children stay in middle of paths, away from tall grass and underbrush?

❏ If outdoors a long time, children are checked periodically for ticks, and again when returning indoors (including neck and scalp)?

Preventing Insect Stings and Bites

❏ Children wear long-sleeved shirts and long pants?

❏ Areas of standing water are drained to prevent mosquito breeding?

❏ Areas around the facility are checked for insect nests to destroy?

❏ Children are kept away from places insects gather, such as garbage cans?

❏ Precautions are taken with children with insect allergies (wear medical ID bracelet, stay away from foods and soft drinks outdoors, not left alone)?

❏ Childcare center policy and parents' wishes are followed for use of repellents? Repellents are used only outdoors, following safety instructions?

Preventing Snakebites

❏ Children are kept away from areas known to have snakes?

❏ If a snake is seen, reverse direction and retrace steps, watching for other snakes?

❏ Children kept from underbrush areas, fallen trees, and other areas where snakes may live?

AUTOMOBILE SAFETY

Motor vehicle crashes are a leading cause of death and injury for children. Use of appropriate car seats is the single most important way to prevent injury. In addition, practice these safe automobile guidelines (**Figure 16-7**):

❏ Child locks are used on rear doors for children under age 6? All doors locked when vehicle is moving?

❏ Young children are not allowed to play with windows? Power windows are kept locked?

❏ Children are taught to exit car on curb side?

❏ Cigarette lighter is removed and disconnected?

❏ Children are never left alone in vehicle?

❏ Vehicle is equipped with a first aid kit and fire extinguisher?

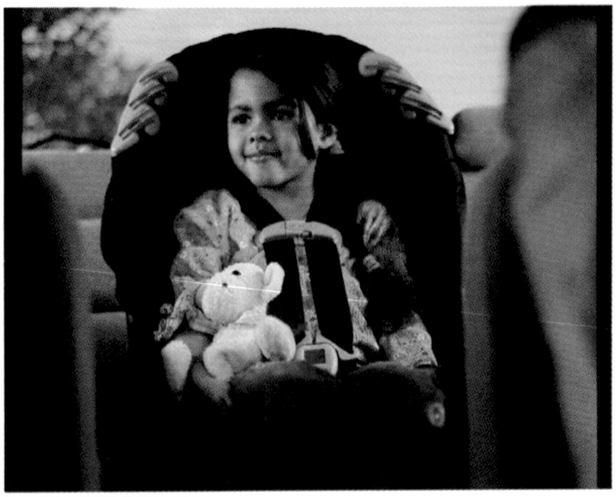

Figure 16-7 Use of appropriate car seats is an important way to prevent injury.

❑ Adults use safety belts for safety and to set an example?

❑ Older children are taught not to get in a vehicle whose driver has been drinking or using drugs?

❑ Only children age 13 or older ride in front seat?

Car Seats and Safety Belts

❑ An approved car seat or belt-positioning booster seat is always used for infants and children?

❑ Automobile and car seat manufacturers' instructions are followed for installation of car or belt-positioning booster seat?

❑ Vehicle back seat is used for car seat? (If front must be used, passenger-side airbag must be disabled.)

❑ Safety seat webbing is always positioned correctly?

❑ Seat is appropriate for size and weight of child?

  ❑ Infants under age 1 and 20–22 lbs should face rear.

  ❑ Infants over age 1 and 20–22 lbs can face forward.

  ❑ Children 40 to 80 lbs (to about age 11) should use a belt-positioning booster seat installed with lap belt and shoulder harness.

❑ Children over 80 lbs use adult belts, with lap belt low and tight across upper thighs and shoulder belt across chest?

WATER SAFETY

❑ Children are never left alone near water? Small children are not left alone in bathtub or wading pool?

❑ Children are not allowed to dive in shallow, murky, or unknown water?

❑ At open waterfronts, children are kept away from areas with big waves, undertows, boats?

❑ Personal flotation devices (life jackets) are used on boats and around water?

❑ Children leave the water if thunder is heard?

❑ In public swimming areas, children enter the water only where lifeguards are present?

❑ Rescue floats and other devices are present at pools and other water areas?

❑ Children at appropriate ages learn to swim from a qualified instructor?

❑ Adult supervisors realize children who can swim are not "drown-proof"?

❑ Adult supervisors are trained in CPR?

❑ Children are never allowed alone on frozen bodies of water?

Index